MIND AND
SUPERMIND

MIND AND SUPERMIND

A *Saturday Review* Report

———— ● ————

Edited by

Albert Rosenfeld

HOLT, RINEHART and WINSTON ● *New York*

Published simultaneously in Canada by Holt, Rinehart
and Winston of Canada, Limited.

Library of Congress Cataloging in Publication Data

Main entry under title:
Mind and supermind.

   "Originally appeared in issues of *Saturday Review.*"
   Bibliography: p.
   Includes index.
   1. Consciousness. 2. Brain. 3. Psychotherapy.
I. Rosenfeld, Albert. II. Saturday review.
BF311.M55   153   76–29912
ISBN 0–03–018961–6

Designer: Kathy Peck

Printed in the United States of America
10 9 8 7 6 5 4 3 2 1

All articles in this volume originally appeared in issues
of *Saturday Review.*

"In God's Image" from *The Ultimate Athlete,* copyright © 1975
by George Leonard, reprinted by permission of The Viking Press,
Inc.

CONTENTS

Introduction by Albert Rosenfeld   ix

Part One: Expanding the Limits of Consciousness

Introduction, *by Albert Rosenfeld*   3
In God's Image, *by George Leonard*   7
Putting the First Man on Earth,
   by Jean Houston   15
The Psychophysical Experience,
   by Robert Masters   27
Biofeedback: An Exercise in
   "Self-Control," *by Barbara Brown*   34
The Consciousness Revolution,
   by John W. White   47
   Afterword: A Layman's Guide to the
      World of PSI, *by John W. White*   57
Mind-and-Supermind in Science Fiction,
   by Isaac Asimov and Ben Bova   62

Part Two: Inside the Brain

Introduction, *by Albert Rosenfeld and
   Kenneth A. Klivington*   77
A Layman's Guide to the Brain, *by Albert
   Rosenfeld and Kenneth A. Klivington*   82
   Afterword: Psychochemistry of the Brain
      by Richard Restak   88

v

Speak, Memory: The Riddle of Recall and
Forgetfulness, *by Maya Pines*　　　　　　90
José Delgado: Exploring Inner Space,
by Richard Restak　　　　　　101
Brain Damage: A Window on the Mind,
by Howard Gardner　　　　　　112
Left-Brain, Right-Brain,
by Roger W. Sperry　　　　　　124
Afterword:　Eyes Left! Eyes Right!
by James H. Austin　　　　　　133
Observing the Brain Through a Cat's Eyes,
by Roger Lewin　　　　　　137
Afterword:　How Real Is Our Reality?
by Albert Rosenfeld　　　　　　144
The Promise and Peril of Psychosurgery,
by Richard Restak　　　　　　148
Afterword:　The Need Is to Know More,
Not Less, *by Albert Rosenfeld*　　　　　　159
Irving Cooper: Pacemakers for the Brain,
by David Hendin　　　　　　162

Part Three:　The Spectrum of Psychotherapy

Introduction, *by Albert Rosenfeld*　　　　　　177
The Psychotherapy Marketplace,
by Morris B. Parloff　　　　　　181
Afterword:　Is Psychiatry a White-
Middle-Class Invention? *by Ari Kiev*　　　　　　195
Toward a Science of the Passions,
by Jarl Dyrud　　　　　　199
And Now, Preventive Psychiatry,
by Albert Rosenfeld　　　　　　211
The Biochemical Roots of Mental
Illness, *by Seymour S. Kety*　　　　　　215
The New Orthomolecular Therapy,
by Joann Rodgers　　　　　　227
Medicine for Melancholy,
by Anthony Wolff　　　　　　237
Can Psychiatry Save the Republic?
by Arthur Schlesinger, Jr.　　　　　　246

CONTENTS

Envoi: *An Editorial by Norman Cousins*   261

Appendixes

Appendix A: Consciousness Research,
What and Where, *by John W. White*   267
Appendix B: A Sampler of Recent Books,
1973–1976   273

Index   285

Introduction
—— • ——
by Albert Rosenfeld

Mind, however we define it, itself defines our humanity. This realization is largely what motivates our pursuit of mind's mysteries with a persistence that borders on the addictive.

The mind of our species probably could not have come into being without the prior advent of certain physiological capacities. We had to develop the opposable thumb in order to grasp and manipulate things. We had to attain the upright position to leave our hands and arms free for tasks other than mere locomotion. Binocular vision and our unique linguistic apparatus were other factors likely to have accompanied the rapid growth (remarkably rapid, on an evolutionary time scale) of the brain, and especially of its convoluted cortex— now seen to be the seat of intelligence and reason.

Whatever our individual persuasion in regard to how we arrived at our status as *Homo sapiens,* we tend to associate mind with the purely *im*material aspects of our existence: thought, intellect, spirit, psyche, personality, character, identity, consciousness, imagination—all the qualities that we can name but not point to; that we know intuitively and subjectively though they cannot be weighed, measured, or experienced via our senses. We think of mind as separate, in its very essence, from the body (including the brain), from the organism so undeniably made of the earthstuff that relates us so intimately to both the animal and the inanimate worlds.

Descartes envisioned the mind (the thinking substance, as he termed it) and the body (the extended, material substance) as two discrete entities running along parallel time tracks, though perfectly synchronized by the strategically located pineal gland—the "third eye" of Oriental religious lore. Modern philosophers, at least since Husserl, have spoken of mind as being "embodied."

The distinguished British neurobiologist the late Sir Russell Brain said flatly that the matter—the atoms and molecules—that makes up the brain, and the mind that results from the organization of that matter, constitute a unity, however separately we might think of them. He suggested that we might have to "leave to the philosophers, who have separated them in thought, the task of putting them together again." And philosophers have labored to comply. The young American philosopher H. Tristram Engelhardt, Jr., for one, views the relation of mind and body "no longer as the association of two substances, two things, but as the integration of two levels of conceptual richness."

Many scientific investigators of mind-body phenomena have come to believe that we cope successfully with the world, as individuals, to the extent that we are able to integrate, in our own lives, these "two levels of conceptual richness."

This is meant to be a practical book. And while it lays no claim to being a complete compendium of current knowledge in the fields of mind, brain, and psychotherapy, it is much more than a random collection of magazine pieces.

These articles, most of which appeared in 1975 and 1976 (though a few go back as far as 1973), reflect an abiding interest in these subjects on the part of *Saturday Review*'s editors; not only the science editor, but also senior editor Hallowell Bowser, managing editor Peter Young (the title *Mind and Supermind* was his brainchild), and of course editor Norman Cousins himself. But they also reflect what we believe to be an abiding interest on the part of our readers.

We live in an age of great confusion. Amid its bewildering complexities we are often unsure of our identities, of what our values are—or ought to be. We are filled with fears and anxieties, and often submerge our hopes in a fraudulent cynicism, yet reach eagerly for any promise of instant self-help or overnight transformation. Meanwhile, there is an explosion of new knowledge from accelerated research in laboratories around the world—not only intensive research on the brain and in the more conventional neurosciences, but also explorations into the more extensive territories of "mind" and "consciousness," variously defined, including some areas that, not long ago, would have been relegated to the fuzzy realms of mysticism. One is reminded of the late Alfred Adler's definition of mysticism as "any science that scientists do not understand." Whenever mystical insights can be encompassed and validated by science, we all stand to benefit—though we must be careful lest, in our eagerness to acquire the presumed benefits, we accept validation too uncritically.

The three parts of this book are taken essentially from three carefully planned special sections of *SR:* "Mind and Supermind" (February 22, 1975), from which the book's title is taken; "Inside the Brain" (August 9, 1975); and "The Psychotherapy Jungle" (February 21, 1976).

In putting these together, we of course knew that, in the present state of knowledge, we would often come up not with simple answers but rather with more complicated questions. As one example of our suspicion borne out, take the heredity vs. environment issue. Almost any broad discussion of human development and behavior will, sooner or later, work around to an argument as to which factor—heredity or environment—is more influential in the formation of individual character. Can brain research shed any light on this controversy? Of course it can.

Dr. Roger Sperry, in his article on the two halves of the brain, believes he has convincingly demonstrated that brain structure and function are considerably *more* dictated by the individual's genetic heritage, and considerably *less* malleable by environmental factors, than was formerly believed. On the other hand, Dr. José Delgado—like Sperry, a pioneering brain researcher—holds the conviction (see Dr. Richard Restak's article about him) that the brain is much more exquisitely subject to environmental influences than anyone has previously imagined. Which of the two experts can we believe? Who is right?

They both are. Instead of a simple answer, we have gained insight into the complexity of the question. We tend to think of heredity and environment as if they were opposite, or at least incompatible, entities; as if we had a limited space into which the two might fit, and if there is more than one then there must be less of the other. And we discover, instead, that we have room for more of both!

We also knew, in assigning and assembling this material, that we could not possibly provide anything like exhaustive coverage of topics so vast in scope. What we tried to do is perhaps best described in radio-engineering jargon: to separate the signals from the noise. In all these subject areas, the public has been assailed on all sides by indigestible masses of information and misinformation, an overload of conflicting input, resulting in what Benjamin DeMott has so concisely characterized as "the stink of hard-sell competition for the troubled soul's buck." How to sort one's way out of the confusion?

These special sections, then, while intended as updated scientific reports that would be intrinsically fascinating, were also calculated to serve as guides for the bedeviled consumer, insofar as such guidance could be offered. Did we succeed? The contents of these issues have received official sanction of a sort, in that they have been used as supplementary reading in a number of college courses and have won awards from organizations as diverse as the National Society for Medical Research and the American Psychological Foundation.

But, even more important, they also struck a chord of recognition in our mass audience of intelligent and curious readers. These issues of the magazine were all best sellers at the newsstand; in fact, "Mind and Supermind" sold out entirely and has for some time been a collector's item. Our mail response was unusually large, even for *SR*'s responsive readers. Letters came in by the hundreds, not only to the magazine but to the individual authors—pleas for help and requests for further information; invitations to lecture, teach, write other articles or books; and commentaries, criticisms, and suggestions of every stripe.

Most letters to the magazine were laudatory and expressed gratitude for filling a felt need. There were plenty of critical letters, too—but the criticism usually was not of what we had said but rather of what we had left out. We had given too-short shrift to some favorite person or therapy, or had omitted some aspect of brain research or psychiatry. Why, some complained, so little attention to R. D. Laing and the *anti*psychiatry movement? Why such passing mention of *est* and TM, when they surely deserved full articles of their own? How come no more than a glance in the direction of Carlos Castaneda's don Juan? Why no full treatment of hypnosis? Why no mention, in the sections on psychopharmacology, of the drug diphenylhydantoin (Dilantin), the anticonvulsant that the Dreyfus Medical Foundation has investigated for a variety of emotional, and especially depressive, disorders? Should we not, in discussing the psychophysiological experience, have spent some time on the "zen of sport" movement that began with a revival of interest in Eugen Herrigel's *Zen in the Art of Archery* and peaked (in the American consciousness, at least) after the publication of W. Timothy Gallwey's *The Inner Game of Tennis*—the movement, exemplified by the work of people like Michael Murphy and George Leonard at the Esalen Institute, in the spiritual and mental aspects of athletics?

One could go on. We knew at the outset that there was no conceivable way our authors could even so much as mention everything, let alone give everyone's favorite topic equal space and time. We did not try to dictate to the writers, many of whom are recognized authorities in their own fields, precisely what they should include within the boundaries of their subject matter, nor what they should emphasize and what they should not. The final results, though far from perfect, did on the whole accomplish our purpose, and did attract a gratifying quantity of favorable attention and comment.

We have left the sections very much as they were originally published in the magazine, though several of the authors exercised their option to revise and update; in no case were the changes extensive. We omitted a few of the very short pieces that seemed not to fit the context of this book. And we did decide to add—in order to enrich our mix and round out our treatment of these topics—a number of articles that had run in other issues of the magazine. These range all the way from the

Asimov–Bova article on science fictional treatment of the themes of mind and brain, to Arthur Schlesinger's provocative commentary on psychiatry as the potential guardian of presidential sanity. They also include articles on brain surgery and psychosurgery; and the distinction between the two is worth emphasizing: brain operations undertaken to repair known brain damage or to remove brain tumors, for instance, are a part of conventional neurosurgery and relatively noncontroversial; psychosurgery, on the other hand, deals specifically with those operations performed for the purpose of controlling *behavioral* disorders, and is an area superheated by ongoing controversy.

Meanwhile, investigation in all these areas surges ahead. Even as I write this introduction, I am looking at a just-opened invitation to an international symposium, sponsored by the National Foundation–March of Dimes, to be held at the University of Texas Medical Branch in Galveston, its participants including a number of Scandinavians, Russians, and Israelis, on "The Immunological Aspects of Schizophrenia." The *immunological* aspects of schizophrenia? *Are* there any? The news is that there are, although the field is too new to fit the preliminary findings into any coherent pattern. And I pick up a copy of *Science* that tells of rapidly accelerating research into the nature of "endorphins," substances naturally made by our own bodies that mimic the effects of morphine and other narcotics—a brand new and exciting branch of neurobiology—and I make a mental note to assign an article on the subject for *SR*.

Then too, I thumb through the most recently arrived issue of *Psychology Today* and stop at a review of a trio of just-published psychiatry books; the review, in essence, laments the absence of any book that gives a comprehensive and well-balanced overview of the subject for the general reader. We do not pretend that this volume fills the vacancy as *the* book that tells all about the subjects of mind, brain, and psychotherapy. But, in all immodesty, we suspect that it comes as close to it as is presently available.

—NEW ROCHELLE, NEW YORK
OCTOBER 1976

PART ONE

•

Expanding the Limits of Consciousness

Introduction

by Albert Rosenfeld

The frontier territories they explore bear such names as the New Consciousness, Mind Research, the Human Potential. The designations vary—and though they are often similar in sound, they are certainly not synonymous. Some of the explorers prefer to carry out their adventurous sorties single-handedly; others go in groups. Their activities are seldom coordinated; in fact, they are often at odds with one another. Yet their territories overlap, and their paths often intersect.

Despite their lack of consensus either in theory or in practice, these investigators all represent related aspects of a ground-swelling movement that is grandiose in its scope, exuberant and evangelistic in its style and tone. Out of this grab bag of diversity somehow has grown a worldwide movement, held together in a directional thrust, as if by a kind of "field energy" made up of common interests and enthusiasms, parallel themes and purposes, and a shared sense of urgency. Books about these explorers often carry titles like *Supernature* and *Supersenses*. Indeed, what they are in quest of might fairly be described as "supermind." Their major goal is to expand human awareness, to convince us that we are greater

3

than we think we are—as great as we will let ourselves become.

The mind they speak of is, in their view, an integrated unity. It is body-brain, psyche-soma, matter-spirit. Even our surroundings are envisioned as part of the self. The world is in a mess, they remind us, and time is short; and the solutions to our problems may lie within ourselves. Hence, the emphasis on inner space rather than outer (except for the school of "ufology" that believes we will be saved, if at all, by the intervention of extraterrestrial beings who pilot or control UFOs). Such are the themes that run through the essays, articles, and reports that make up this section.

We make no pretense at providing exhaustive or definitive coverage of this vast and fuzzy-bordered subject. Nor do we attempt to pass judgment on the claims made by the various movements. But because the larger movement of which they are parts is fascinating in itself; because it is so energetic, so widespread, and of such potential importance; and because we live in an era when the human species needs all the help it can get, from whatever source—for these good reasons we feel the reading public should be acquainted with at least the broad outlines of this new consciousness movement, as presented by some of its participants. The fact that we present a particular theory does *not* necessarily mean that we endorse all that it represents. That would in any case be premature.

Some parts of the new consciousness movement—biofeedback is one example—are already well within the bounds of validated science. Other areas—such as those that make use of altered states of consciousness (ASCs) to promote human awareness and growth—are on their way to gaining acceptance into the family of behavioral sciences. Yet other aspects of the movement—certain facets of psi, for instance—may never be confirmed scientifically, perhaps because they simply may not be amenable to investigation via the traditional scientific method. If even a small part is validated, however, beyond a reasonable doubt, then the effect on our thinking and our behavior may be profound.

The news is that many bona fide, faultlessly credentialed scientists have opened up their minds—and, more important, their labs—to areas of research that they would formerly have considered out of bounds, if not downright nonsense. A word of caution is called for here: The mere opening of the mind to a possibility does not constitute acceptance or proof. Many scientists, after they have taken a hard look at some of the claimed data, may well conclude that what they used to think of as nonsense is *still* nonsense. But there is much less likelihood of an unconsidered brush-off in an age when Yogic powers—for example, the power to slow one's heartbeat at will—have been verified in the lab, when at least some aspects of acupuncture have proved medically valid, and when a major university (U.C.L.A.) awards a graduate degree to a sorcerer's apprentice (Carlos Castaneda).

Because science has for so long ignored their favorite areas of research, many in the "psi" or "human potential" movement still find themselves reflexively attacking Establishment science. Yet some among them are as closed-minded as they have ever accused science of being. To criticize science for its past and continuing lack of interest is one thing. But to take the attitude "Okay, if you won't believe my facts, I won't believe yours either" is to cut oneself off from much of the world's soundest and hardest-won knowledge and is thus foolish and counterproductive. It has taken a long time to win science's cautious interest in what amounts to a union with myth, mysticism, and metaphysics. This interest could be all too easily turned off. That would be a pity. The new presence in the movement of established science, with its experimental competence and its built-in skepticism, is good and reassuring news.

From the viewpoint of traditional science, the worst that can happen if we give the "mind sciences" an open hearing is that some time and energy will have been wasted (though entertainingly). What is unacceptable simply will not be accepted. On the other hand, if any *new* discoveries are made (or old ones validated) that might help us surmount our proliferating problems—whether in terms of personal values or global ecologies—we will all be the grateful beneficiaries.

In God's Image
•
by George Leonard

Only a few years ago futurists were making wildly enthusiastic claims for an imminent golden age of computers. In 1968, for example, Herman Kahn of the Hudson Institute foresaw that the extensive use of computerized robots to help with housework and other chores would be "very likely" by the year 2000; he called it an even bet that true artificial intelligence would be developed by then. Arthur C. Clarke's book—and the movie derived from it—of the late sixties, *2001: A Space Odyssey,* gave us an unforgettable hero and villain, Hal the Computer, who not only understood and spoke perfect idiomatic English but also could pick up subtle nuances of intonation. Although I conceived of the CAD (Computer Assisted Dialogue) in my *Education and Ecstasy* independently of Clarke's work, it shared some of Hal's capabilities, along with—*mea culpa*—humor and an aesthetic sense.

Without much thought on the matter, we came to accept computers and other technological devices as

George Leonard is the author of *Education and Ecstasy, The Transformation,* and *The Ultimate Athlete,* from which this article is adapted.

superhuman. In television cartoons and science fiction thrillers, the computer, the robot, and the cyborg (a combination of living organism and machine) took on the role of *deus ex machina*—the all-knowing, all-powerful god of our age. The popularization of the man-machine linkup reached a new low, I believe, in the television series "The Six-Million-Dollar Man," in which a badly injured astronaut has been rebuilt as part man, part computerized machinery. The resulting cyborg, television's candidate for the Ultimate Athlete, possesses superhuman powers of strength, speed, agility, and perception. These powers are usually dedicated to the pursuit of unpleasant criminal types in episodes just as seedy and dehumanizing as those presented on any other crime show.

In the sober light of the mid-seventies, it now appears that both futurists and popularizers have been premature in their assessment. Computers can indeed perform certain feats of computation and retrieval that seem to be beyond normal human mental powers. We are finding out, however, that even the largest, most advanced computer cannot be made to understand sentences that a four-year-old child can comprehend without hesitation. And so simple a trick as riding a bicycle without using the hands has thus far resisted duplication by sophisticated space-age technology: A NASA-sponsored bicycle-balancing robot recently failed to do what any twelve-year-old would gladly demonstrate. Right now, in fact, the development of a simple household robot, much less a Hal or a Six-Million-Dollar Man, seems more remote than it did eight or ten years ago.

What we are learning is not that computers are any less wonderful than we had imagined but that human abilities are far more wonderful than we had dreamed. When we set about programming computers to understand a simple sentence, we were forced to realize the tremendous number of logical steps, the brilliant inferences, and the vast body of knowledge necessary for a process that we had previously just taken for granted. And until we attempted to make a robot that could ride a bicycle without using its hands, we had not properly appreciated the superb balance and control involved in some of our most mundane acts. The Age of Computers may indeed turn out to be golden after all, if only because it reveals to us the miracle inherent in what we consider most ordinary in our lives.

Confronted daily with the failure of human beings to get along with one another, with the seemingly fatal flaws in our social systems, and with the pathogenic despair and cynicism of our arts and entertainment, we often find it easy to be pessimistic about human prospects. But that pessimism cannot explain why we continually overlook the potential of our species, the awesome capacities of all life on this planet, the even more awesome capabilities of human consciousness. It is as if it would be too painful to face the truth, to look into that great chasm between what we are and what we could be. Fearing the brightness of our own potentialities, we keep watching the shadows on the wall of the cave, calling the larger vision "unscientific," "soft." But even that rationalization is being taken away from us. Modern physics comes ever more closely to resemble the Perennial Philosophy; already it is impossible, as research psychologist Lawrence LeShan demonstrates, to distinguish statements by famous physicists from those by great mystics. And even the hardest science is now corroborating the vision of life, body, and mind that the cynics would call soft.

We find it easy to imagine superhuman robots, but now science is showing us that our own abilities are even more remarkable. For example, recent experiments by Dr. Barbara Sakitt, a physicist-psychologist now at Stanford University, have shown that the unaided human eye can detect a *single quantum* of light—that is, the smallest amount of energy possible in our known universe. The

9

quantum is a unit of energy so small that the energy a piece of chalk releases when falling one-thousandth of an inch would be 1 trillion quanta. Then, too, we find it easy to be dumbfounded by the amount of information that can be stored in an advanced computer, until we begin to consider that a single ordinary-sized gene can be arranged in some 10^{600} different ways. (To get an idea of the magnitude of this number, you might bear in mind that the entire universe contains only an estimated 10^{80} atoms.) A gene is made of DNA, the basic blueprint for all life as we know it. A virus, the simplest form of life, consists of a gene or genes with a protein cover. Thus, it may be said that the world of viruses, submicroscopic entities so small that they will pass through most filters, has informational possibilities that would stagger the largest computer.

But let us expand our imagination from viruses to a single human being with 100,000 or more genes and with trillions of individual cells arranged in any number of complex patterns. And let us focus for a moment on that particular concentration of information-carrying cells or neurons called the brain, and on all the multifarious interactions of those neurons—the complex pathways of synapses, the domains of cooperating neurons, the pulse of the information-carrying waves, the constant, flickering electrochemical changes within and between neurons, the information-multiplying capacities between brain and "mind," the constant interplay between areas of the brain and every muscle, organ, nerve, and sensory receptor in the body. Let us focus also on the interplay between all of this and what is outside the skin, with nature and culture, and perhaps with zones of information we have not yet identified. Indeed, the number of possible interactions within the brain alone is beyond the current skill of our best mathematicians to compute in a meaningful manner. The best way of expressing the total creative capacity of the human central nervous system in layman's language is to say that for all practical purposes it is infinite.

Thus, science brings us around to a central thesis of most of the world's religions, a subtle and profound mystery in the *Brahma Sutra,* and a single spine-tingling sentence in the King James version of the Bible: "So God created man in His own image, in the image of God He created him; male and female created He them."

In God's image! How could we possibly live up to such a pronouncement? We take comfort in the fact that our religions also concede that we are fallen, unsaved, unenlightened. No matter how fallen, however, we can no longer deny our godlike capacities—science will not permit the denial. And we are reminded of the ancient religious promise: the ultimate availability of salvation, redemption, transformation.

If we find any truth in this argument about man's capacities, we are forced to regard our present life with a certain wonder and bewilderment. It is not just war and disease and famine and obvious social injustice that appall us; it is also the pervasive waste of human potential. Aware of man's godlike capacities, we see individual lives dedicated to rudimentary, deadening, demeaning pursuits. Aware of transcendent possibilities in everyday activities, we see our best and brightest people attracted to cold, insensitive manipulation on the one hand and trivial quasi-artistic fads on the other. And we see God's image grubbing and grabbing for meaningless consumer products. Waste!

When speaking of human potential, we must make certain qualifications. Not all of it can be used for creation and enlightenment. Many of the circuits in our body and brain must be redundant in order for life to persist. Some of our capacities must be devoted to low-order survival needs. And as we create higher levels of order, we must also deal with inevitable disorder. But even after we have made these provisos, it is still clear that we are operating with only a tiny fraction of our true abilities. Studying nature, we find that systems are created to be used to the full. What is the purpose of all the unused human capability? What is its destination?

In our search for answers, we have been blinded by both the past and the future, by "history" and "the year 2000." "History" tells us that human nature does not change. But history is the record of events only since the beginning of civilization—that is, about the time of the Pyramid Age. The entire period we know as history has been based on a single major organizational mode, built around the problem of dealing with the agricultural surplus that accumulated from the successful large-scale cultivation of grain crops. This surplus resulted in the development of markets, legalism, caste and class; the construction of pyramids, cathedrals, high-rise buildings, communications networks, swift vehicles, huge military machines; the growth of cities, nations, and empires. Individual consciousness, insofar as possible, was fixed and limited. Mind was separated from body. The vast majority of human beings were used as standardized components in the social machine. More and more energy was harnessed. More and more matter was controlled. The human potential was not the major factor in the equation.

Looking backward to prehistory and forward beyond the year 2000, we realize that the period designated as history actually constitutes only one brief segment of the larger human journey. In my book *The Transformation* I outlined the earlier transformations (from primitive hunting-and-gathering band to tribal village, from tribal village to civilized state) that led to the current period, detailed the characteristics of the epoch of civilization, and argued that a major transformation into something quite different is already under way. Since the publication of that book in 1972, it has become increasingly apparent that the current major mode of social organization is no longer tenable. In the light of present realities, time-honored principles of economics, agriculture, education, and social control are revealed as clearly faulty. Individual alienation increases at an alarming rate. The entire social structure, with all its mighty physical works, now appears to us somehow fragile and vulnerable.

Clearly, some great change is under way. We might have seen it earlier had technological futurism not seduced us. The year 2000, which turns out to have been merely a strategy for justifying "the same, only more so," has kept us from seeing the present, where a transformation is already occurring. We should have known that all along. Existence is not fixed; even the mightiest social organism eventually evolves into something else. This evolution means the death of old forms but does not necessarily mean the catastrophic death of individual human beings. Still, at this moment, the odds on a relatively peaceful transformation seem rather long. We face the possibility of physical catastrophe along with the breakdown of old forms in the absence of new. We face the possibility of variations on the theme of a police state as social leaders react to the rise of anarchic tendencies. But we also face the possibility—it would be both cowardly and illogical simply to dismiss it—of a less-dreadful change, in which our enormous untapped potential would be used to the full: long odds, enormous difficulties, miracles!

Some sort of transformation is inevitable in any case. The present social machinery can probably be glued together and heated up a few more times, at least in nations as wealthy as the United States. But each year brings us closer to the realization that our present way of doing and being cannot last very much longer. If our shift to a new mode of existence is to take place voluntarily, before catastrophe strikes, we shall need to get on with the business of converting our energy-economic system from exponential growth to something approaching a steady state, a process that itself will require great amounts of energy. The resulting economic dislocation must be dealt with equitably, with a sense of sacrifice—especially on the part of the affluent.

Sacrifice, however, requires some guiding purpose and, ideally, some notion of better things to come. It is doubtful that purely negative exhortations can inspire the great efforts needed for the survival of a humane social order. Dismayed by the prospect of long-term reduction in our material standard of living, we need a clearer vision of how it feels to be alive. This vision may at last draw us to the most plentiful resource on this planet: our own unused capacities. The human brain, the most complex entity in the known universe, has not necessarily evolved merely to aid in the production and consumption of ever more trivial goods and services. Perhaps this complex and marvelous entity can help us turn to other kinds of wealth—nonmaterial wealth—and other kinds of energy—the energy of the spirit, which burns no fuel, depletes no resources, and creates no pollution. Perhaps we shall eventually realize that changes in the nature of what is rewarding to human individuals must accompany reforms in politics, health care, defense and foreign policy, law, justice, and human rights.

But our hope lies not in the brain alone or in the mind alone, but rather in mind, body, and spirit rejoined. (How could we ever have conceived of them as separate?) This resource is close at hand, readily available, crying out to be used. In material shortages and social difficulties, even in what we term economic depression, we may find clues to the next chapter in the human adventure: the evolution of higher social forms, the emergence of a higher consciousness.

Putting the First
Man on Earth
•
by Jean Houston

In our laboratory at the Foundation for Mind Research (FMR), a pianist is put into a light trance state
by simple verbal suggestion. As she goes deeper into
trance, she is instructed to practice a sonata that she
must soon perform at a concert. It is a piece she
knows well but has not played in a long while. She is
now told to take all the time she needs for perfecting
the piece. Upon emerging from the trance, she says
she feels much more confident after an intensive hour
of rehearsal. So saying, she sits down at the piano and
demonstrates how much her playing of the sonata has
indeed improved.

Two remarkable things have happened. The improvement took place even though the pianist had only *imagined* the rehearsal session. Yet the exercise had done her
as much good as if she had actually practiced on a real
piano. The other, and perhaps more remarkable, aspect
of the experiment: Though she subjectively had a good

Dr. Jean Houston is the director of the Foundation for Mind Research and
co-author with her husband, Dr. Robert Masters, of *The Varieties of Psychedelic
Experience* and *Mind Games.*

hour's practice, in fact only one minute of "real" clock time had passed!

How to explain these phenomena?

We freely admit how incomplete our present understanding is. But while others explore the neurophysiological pathways in the hope of pinpointing the precise mechanisms, we can make some good guesses. Athletes, astronauts, and Yogis have long known that this technique works—that some little-understood "ideomotor" reflexes exist by which the mere *thinking* of an action can somehow signal the involved muscles to respond, albeit imperceptibly. This phenomenon was known to the late F. Matthias Alexander, whose psychophysical theories so profoundly influenced such thinkers as John Dewey and George Bernard Shaw; it is even better known to the contemporary genius of psychophysical engineering, Israel's Moshe Feldenkrais. But the action practiced in the imagination *must be known to the body from past experience.* It won't help to imagine that you're playing a sonata or hitting a tennis ball if you've never done these things. And the "imagining" must transcend our usual lazy imagining; it must be concentrated and powerfully evocative —a total *mind-body visualization* of the act.

But what of the time-compression effect that enabled the pianist to do an hour's subjective practice in only a minute of objective time? Here again, the precise neural mechanisms are not yet known. But we do know that in an altered state of consciousness, such as the trance state represents, we can bypass purely *linear* time—where events proceed step by chronological step as though narrated in verbal sequences. Again, the mind-body visualization process somehow integrates the experience into an accelerated mental process (AMP). In fiction we often read about a character's whole life unfolding before him in a split instant before death. This phenomenon is now corroborated by data collected over a period of time by members of the Swiss Alpine Club, from climbers who,

16

believing their death was imminent, underwent exactly such experiences.

Let me cite one more striking example from our own lab: A songwriter in a trance is told to wander into an imaginary café in a distant city where she will hear an imaginary singer singing songs she has never heard before. She does so, in accelerated time. When she is out of the trance, we ask her what happened—and, as part of her account, she spends fifteen minutes singing a pleasant and original number and portions of two others. We are not suggesting that she was teleported to some strange other world to hear these new songs—only that her creative capacities had been somewhat enhanced so the process could take place.

This creative potential is only one of a whole range of capacities that may be tapped—and tapped not only for officially "creative" artists but also for ordinary people everywhere; and this is what gives the greatest excitement to our quest. In an era when our nation has spent billions of dollars and made prodigious efforts in an astronaut program designed to put the first man on the moon, we now propose a "psychenaut" program, the aim of which is to *put the first man on Earth.*

Though my phrasing is whimsical, the goal is by no means frivolous. Billions of men and women have lived and died here, true enough, since *Homo* first became *sapiens.* But we at FMR, in growing agreement with other explorers along the same frontiers, have come to believe that never in history has there lived on this planet—with perhaps the rarest individual exceptions—the person who has attained his true potential as a whole human being. This is the more aware, more realized human being we seek to put on Earth.

The psychenaut program would be an exploration of

---

*In 1969, Dr. Joel Elkes of Johns Hopkins suggested a somewhat similar "intronaut" program.

inner space. It would map the mind and tap its unrealized capacities. It would acquaint the psychenauts with the phenomenal contents of their own beings—their mind-body systems—and teach them to employ and to enjoy the multiplicity of human qualities that seem almost unattainable on first encounter. Through intensive training, psychenauts would have new control over their creative energies, their health, their experiences of time and space, heat and cold, pain and pleasure.

This exploration of the farther reaches of human consciousness typifies a new kind of mind research, already well begun. Scientists, psychologists, and technicians of every stripe are gathering together with priests, shamans, mystics, artists, madmen, healers, and Yogis, in conferences, academic seminars, laboratories, and ashrams, in a curious blending and interchange of ancient gnosis with contemporary know-how. The result is a strange yeasting of East and West, science and ritual, the distant past and the emergent future. The science of man is thus becoming much richer than what we used to call psychology.

As we conduct this research, we are of course in for surprises, because much of our mind-body system remains a mystery. But many of the "new" capacities have really been known and used for centuries. There has simply never before been a major systematic effort to harness them on a large scale. The idea is not to develop a handful of supermen whom the many will admire. Rather will the program be designed *for* the many. Only a few astronauts could hope to reach the moon, but the psychenauts who finally arrive on Earth could well number in the millions. All authenticated discoveries—and rediscoveries—would be democratized by incorporating them into the educational process at the earliest stages of life.

Look at the life of the average person today, even in the most enlightened and affluent nations. Already in early childhood, a crippling of the physical (though never *purely* physical) person begins at the most fundamental levels. (See Robert Masters's piece on page 27.) Meanwhile, society sanctions the shackling of the mind and the placing of blinders on consciousness. Out of the broad spectrum of possible states of consciousness, we lock ourselves (and one another) into a recognition of only a narrow range of states that we then call "normal." This narrow band might be termed the "cultural trance" —that is, those visions of reality that a given culture permits. Thus we limit our experience, dilute (even at times deny altogether) many of our natural capacities, and effectively prevent the emergence of our full humanity.

Our image of ourselves may be largely to blame. Until very recently our dominant self-image was that of *homo laborans,* man the worker. The man who defines and discovers himself exclusively in terms of what he does in order to put food in his mouth and to maintain a roof overhead becomes proficient in only those skills and potentials that enable him to subsist. His vision narrows, and he dissociates himself from his own body as well as from the body of nature. He lives to manipulate. And he looks outside himself for the fulfillment of his needs.

We have not changed much in this respect since prehistory. Our sophisticated technology is in many ways merely an extension of the ax, the stone, and the spear. We have invented prosthetic extensions of our hands, feet, eyes, and senses, but our primitive materialistic outlook has kept us from discovering—or even looking for —our own innate powers.

Will the psychenauts, then, retreat from the outside world and withdraw into themselves? Not at all. To do so would be self-defeating. It is enormously significant that the current crisis of consciousness—the loss of a sense of reality felt by so many, the rising tide of alienation—occurs concomitantly with the ecological destruc-

19

tion of the planet. We are forced into the realization that a human being is not an encapsulated bag of skin that lives in isolation. He is not only mind-body but also organism-environment. The healthy psychenaut will have to harmonize the inner and outer worlds.

At FMR we have for more than ten years been engaged in a kind of precursor psychenaut program. We have worked with hundreds of research subjects representing a wide sampling of the population. With them we have experimented with the so-called altered and expanded states of consciousness. We have seen the remarkable speeding up of normal mental processes, already mentioned, the control and enhancement of all the senses, the modulation of pain and pleasure. We have learned much about religious and "peak" experiences, about the nature and facilitation of creativity, about the programming and practical uses of dreams. We have investigated some of the phenomena associated with parapsychology. We have been able to impart, through biofeedback training, physiological control of internal and involuntary states. We have learned that the body *can* be reeducated.

From all this and more has emerged the conviction that ordinary people, given the opportunity and training, can come a long way toward attaining their unsuspected potential. Once they can emancipate themselves from a host of anxieties, fears, inhibitions, and outmoded and unflattering images of themselves, they can quickly begin to think, feel, and *know* in genuinely new ways, and to aspire, within realistic limits, to a multidimensional awareness of their mind-bodies and the environmental context in which they are immersed.

Training to restore an integral sense of body-mind comes first. (See again Dr. Masters's piece.) Over a period of weeks, months, and in some cases years, research subjects learn to master these psychophysical procedures and at the same time to experience altered states of consciousness. Breaking through the surface crust of what we ordinarily call consciousness—the "cultural trance"—is all-important to success. The best place to start is outside the range of this "normal" consciousness.

Throughout history some people have known this fact and have invented or discovered many techniques and systems for escaping this limitation; to alter consciousness as a gateway to subjective realities, to heightened sensitivity, to aesthetic and creative apperceptions; and to make consciousness available to religious experience. Ritual drumming, dancing, chanting, fasting, the ingestion of mind-altering plant substances, Yoga and meditative states—these and many other means have been used to suspend the cultural trance so that alternate realities and solutions could be perceived.

We have worked with many of these ancient and "primitive" procedures, employing contemporary counterparts and methodologies, occasionally marrying ancient technique to modern technology. We have also invented or borrowed new instrumentation by which depth probings of the psyche can be accomplished—and capacities that have been blocked can, to an extent, be unfettered and guided experimentally. We have used sensory-deprivation chambers in which the subject, deprived of his usual visual and auditory reference points, begins to hallucinate and projects his own internal visual and auditory structures. This experiment has helped us to study the image-making processes of the mind. Until 1965, when legislation ended most such research, we also experimented with psychedelic drugs, especially LSD.

Stroboscopic lights have enabled us to stimulate ideo-retinal patterns in order to study "eidetic perception" (the images seen when the eyes are closed). We have used and monitored brain-wave, temperature, and muscular responses, self-regulated by means of biofeedback equipment and training. Our lab also houses consciousness-altering devices, including fairly elaborate audiovisual environments and a swinging vertical cradle that induces unusual trance states, called an Altered States of Consciousness Induction Device (ASCID). Often altered states are elicited by purely verbal means, using trance induction, rhythmic exercises, and vocal drama to elicit hyperalert states. (Some subjects, born to technology, cannot seem to respond without gadgetry, but they can usually be weaned away from the machines after a while.)

What are some of the human potentials that we and others in the field are exploring? First, we know, and can readily demonstrate, that the human mind has a natural capacity to think in visual images as well as in words. This trait is especially true of young children. Though our emphasis on verbal processes inhibits this capacity, thus harming the natural visualizers among us, it can be reactivated. In some artists, scientists, mathematicians, and others the inhibition has been less effective. According to his own statement, Einstein accomplished his most important thought with visual and kinesthetic images, not with words or numbers. Other highly creative people have made similar statements, and much evidence indicates that thinking in images may produce solutions and express ideas that purely verbal thinking cannot. Images may be auditory or kinesthetic as well as visual, and they may involve areas of the brain where the thought process is more susceptible to patterns, to symbolic processes, and to constellational constructs. More information is likely to be condensed in the dynamics inherent in the coded symbolic image. The so-called creative breakthroughs might then be seen as the orchestration of these larger patterns of information.

When consciousness is altered and imagery becomes accessible, the images may be controlled or allowed to emerge spontaneously from various levels of the mind. A novelist, then, may observe a chapter of his novel as he might observe a film, tuning in on a creative process

22

that usually reaches his awareness only as words. At deeper levels, what is experienced may be the stuff of myths or a symbolic drama that profoundly reveals the person's needs and nature. Such images, from the deepest levels of the psyche, may also have the character of spiritual visions or of realities that seem universal and eternal.

In most cases, however, the imagery arises from less-profound depths, as naturally as dream images arise in sleep. People learn to question and program this waking-imagery process, and it responds with answers that might not be possible if they relied solely on verbal thought. A scientist may solve a problem this way; in fact, history records many instances of important discoveries first experienced as spontaneous visual images. Almost any kind of problem may be approached—a dancer may visualize a dance in a flash, a student may solve some academic problem, a psychiatrist may hit upon a diagnostic insight.

Completely new knowledge is not gained by this route any more than by verbal thought, but what *is* obtained is usually not reachable by other means. Image thinking is an *alternative way,* and a very fruitful way, of thinking —a natural endowment we lose too often and too early. Education in the future will undoubtedly encourage, train, and apply image thought as routinely as we now use language; the result should be not only enriched imagination and creativity but also better-balanced personalities.

As we have already seen, the imaging process can result in greatly accelerated mental processes. But it is also possible to *de*celerate the mental process. To what end? As one example, an expectant mother was told that when labor pains began, she would experience hours of clock-measured time as just minutes. She was also told that the pains would be minimal or even experienced as pleasurable. Her several hours of labor then seemed to last no more than thirty minutes, and the childbirth proved to be intensely pleasurable. She did not receive an anesthetic, because avoidance of chemical anesthesia was her motive for participating in the experiment.

Experimentally it is often possible to dilute intensity of pain and shorten its experienced duration and, on the other hand, to intensify and prolong pleasure. Some usually undeveloped senses may be educated. A subject may be told, for instance, not only that he can hear music with his ears but also that he can hear it and be touched by it over the entire surface of his body. This realization gives rise to intense pleasure sensations. Moreover, two or three minutes of music may seem to last for hours. The subject may also be introduced to synesthesia (cross-sensing) and told that it is possible to see music, smell it, taste it—to experience it with all his senses. This is frequently the most powerful and beautiful musical experience the person has ever had. With practice, the new way of responding to music can be extended to experiencing other things in life in expanded and cross-sensory ways until they become natural and ordinary.

Pleasure sensations and aesthetic enjoyment may also be enhanced by removing conceptual blocks to perception—especially early teachings about the inferiority of matter and negative attitudes about the body. In altered states the sanctioning of pleasure can serve to overcome the blocks that culture has imposed. This is especially important for older people who, in America, undergo a progressive lowering of sensory acuity. They cannot see, hear, touch, or use any of their senses *as well as their true physical capacity allows.* This neglect is due as much to our cultural attitudes as to their age. In many tribal and hunting societies, it is the adult, not the child, who is *expected* to evince—and therefore does evince—the most acute and integrated balance of his senses. In our own culture we have the evidence of those professionals who have to keep up a certain sensory acuity for the sake of their art

—the musician's ear, the artist's eye, the *parfumeur*'s nose.

All this argument barely suggests the potential that large numbers of people could actualize in the near future, given the training. Yet, consider how utopian the list sounds to contemporary ears, which accept all sorts of needless limitations just because they pertain to an image of man that we have not seriously challenged.

First of all, the attainable goal is a human being who understands the possibilities of consciousness across the entire broadened spectrum of reality. This psychenaut may orchestrate the movements of his body with high grace and rare efficiency and also may control his internal bodily functions to the degree that those in remote Himalayan retreats do. By working with some of the techniques and states of consciousness described in this article as well as with biofeedback training, and using them routinely in schools, children will learn such self-controls. Pain will still be needed as a warning, but we may not need to suffer it otherwise or to resort to anesthetics to allay it. Pleasure can be enhanced and extended and our perceptual windows regularly cleansed and cross-linked so that one can hear color and see sound, touch taste and smell music.

The "first man on Earth" will relax or alert himself as he chooses. Keeping warm in cold weather, or cool in hot, may be no problem. Dreams and other states could be used for solving problems and for bringing a wiser and more sensitive consciousness to bear on questions of interpersonal relations. People may range over a great variety of mental states, playing upon the instrument of their mind-body as one currently plays other instruments—so that ecstatic and peak experiences, even those experiences that we call mystical and unitive, may be brought within our reach if we are ready for them. A very large historical literature attests to the therapeutic and growth-promoting—and creativity-inducing—potentials

25

of experiences that have traditionally been described as mystical, transcendental, or part of the "cosmic consciousness." Our research indicates that these potentials are in fact indigenous to the human psyche, natural if nonordinary ways of knowing and being, and that they can be midwived in a congenial setting if the subject is properly prepared.

We have developed a few experimental programs for schools, have used some of our techniques to rehabilitate prisoners, and have trained many professionals in health and education; but our efforts are but tiny rafts in a sea of need. It is impossible to state what man's limitations are. Now, if we dare, we can begin to forge a richer, a more fully human, consciousness, and bring into being a new and unifying image of man—man as a being of great, barely tapped potentials—who by means of these potentials might prevail even now.

The Psychophysical
Experience
—— • ——
by Robert Masters

In the present "normal" course of human development,
even by the end of the third year of life, coordination has
become impaired in most persons. By the time that an
individual has reached his late teens, he is likely to have
marked muscular and postural defects. The body is already twisted and tilted, fewer movements are performed, and some parts of it have assumed rigidly fixed
positions. The individual has lost awareness of the body
image (the body's surface and the joints of the skeletal
structure) to the extent that his actions become more
and more automatic and patterns of muscular tension
have developed of which he has little or no consciousness. Deterioration of posture (the correct positioning of
the body with respect to gravity) means a constant *excessive* expenditure of energy in the performance of everything he does, including even standing and sitting.

Not only ordinary persons but also all but a very few
experts fail to recognize these and other defects. Physi-

Dr. Robert Masters is the director of research at the Foundation for Mind
Research and co-author, with his wife, Dr. Jean Houston, of *The Varieties of
Psychedelic Experience* and *Mind Games*.

cians and physical-education instructors take such changes for granted—when they notice them at all—and lack even a conception of how the human body *ought* to feel, of how it ought to move, and of the extent to which kinesthetic consciousness has been diminished and sensory responsiveness diluted. Only the *exceptional* debility is noted, and the "healthy, well-functioning body" is considered one not crippled by glaring abnormalities.

Such fundamental ignorance is self-perpetuating. We have no way of knowing that our incorrect posture makes our bodies feel heavy and that it is wasteful of energy—unless, with the posture corrected, we then learn by experience that the body feels almost weightless and that movements become smooth and flowing. Until awareness is restored to our bodies, we have no way of knowing that tensions have afflicted the muscles, that our joints have stiffened, and that we customarily move without any awareness of how our most routine actions are performed. Only when we have regained awareness and have experienced our bodies as they ought to function will we be able to determine what is "right" and what is "wrong" in our self-use.

Western medicine and physical education stem from ideologies that have separated mind from body and that, moreover, are more anciently rooted in contempt for the body and matter in relationship to spirit. Western thought has instilled in us a basic, if often unconscious, disparagement of pleasurable feelings and sensations, of awareness in the body, and of basic intentions toward the body that go beyond its maintenance as a dwelling place for mind and as a vehicle for the performance of constructive tasks. Hence, the notion of "health" is limited to states that will not distract mind or interfere with work. Even the training of athletes is aimed at optimizing specific task performance.

The goals of conventional physical education do not aspire beyond giving strength, stamina, and some suppleness to the human body—the three main criteria of fitness recognized by Western systems. These are all worthwhile, if limited, goals, but they ignore the fundamentals of correct body use and the body awareness essential to such use. In practice, most physical training consists of mere mechanical repetition of movements and only a very limited range of movements when the possible range is considered. Such exercise has value only inasmuch as it stimulates circulation and uses the muscles. Because it leaves basic defects uncorrected, actually it strengthens the defects. Most importantly, perhaps, most exercise is boring, strenuous, and typically competitive, so most persons experience it as something unpleasant—almost a kind of punishment. This negative conditioning frequently results in a lifelong aversion to physical exercise, and when it becomes imperative for reasons of health that an adult exercise, the problem of motivation is constant and obstructive.

In adulthood we are prone to the incorrect use of the body, the persistence of tensions and wastes of energy, and negative attitudes toward physical training, all of which are conducive to emotional and physical sickness, premature aging, and, almost certainly, shortening of the life span. The limiting of movement to a few stereotyped actions diminishes the range of activities we engage in. Fatigue, the depletion of energy resources, has similar results. Appearance deteriorates, as does the body, and we acquire a potent orientation to, and acceptance of, aging and death. Physical education, in failing both to teach a body-mind understanding and to motivate people to care for themselves, causes a tragedy of staggering dimensions.

Consideration of this tragedy, along with the desire to apply some of our research findings in the field, led us at the Foundation for Mind Research (FMR) first to a search for already-existing systems, not of physical but rather of *psycho*physical education—that is to say, systems that do not divide the body from the mind or ignore the importance of consciousness, but instead seek to work with the unity of body and mind that constitutes the human person.

Most of the methods approaching that ideal originated centuries ago in the East, where there has been a traditional emphasis upon the study and expansion of consciousness and where the aim has been a positive realization of the body's capacities for sensory experience, for self-regulation of many bodily functions, and for avoiding or delaying what Westerners think of as normal aging processes. The East has created numerous such disciplines, of which Yoga is the most widely known.

Yoga and the various schools of "martial arts" all are much more sophisticated than Western physical education and a great deal more demanding. The Yogi performs more movements, involves more of his body, and his physical action always has *an accompanying mental component.* There is an emphasis on grace and flowing lightness that makes actions pleasurable and so enhances motivation. He achieves so high a degree of body awareness that it becomes possible to eliminate many defects by his own efforts. All these systems have much to offer, and it would be a major research effort to take from them what is best and then achieve a synthesis more effective than any single system.

However, our search led us finally to a method that is more sophisticated and, I believe, better applicable to the needs of contemporary peoples in Western societies. This is the "Method" of Moshe Feldenkrais, an Israeli whose practical knowledge of the mechanics of the living human body probably has never been equaled. Feldenkrais, a doctor of applied physics, has developed more than a thousand elaborate exercises, each with some forty variations, by means of which the human frame can virtually be rebuilt.

The FMR programs are indebted to all these sources

for knowledge and inspiration. However, we have endeavored to develop programs that confer many of the same benefits but that are not so complex and otherwise demanding and may be readily taught to available teachers and thus have the most widespread application possible. Although applicable to all age groups, these programs probably have their most important application in the rehabilitation of the adult. They are suitable for work with groups or by individuals.

In our psychophysical educational system, a pleasure principle is continuously operative. Research subjects perform a very great range of movements—always without strain or insistence upon goals—and utilize diversity as a preventive of boredom. They are encouraged to take pleasure in their bodies and to regard an enhancement of sensory awareness as one of the results to be expected and valued. Exercises are arranged in such a manner as to give a frequent demonstration of increasing capacities —another source of pleasure contributing to positive motivation.

As the training progresses, we provide experience illustrating how the body ought to feel and move—for example, in lengthening and lightening of the body, and in easy, flowing movements, in breathing that is free. Such changes are not retained in the beginning, but they demonstrate in the most convincing way, by immediate experience, what is possible.

With further work, the body becomes more supple than most people would have believed possible. They experience the body as light and almost weightless, and objective measurement verifies that just when it seems lightest it is most strong and able to move most swiftly. As joints are freed, there is an increase in speed, fluidity, and ease of movement. Increasingly, persons establish good coordination so that all relevant parts of the body act together to facilitate all movements; whereas before, some parts of the body remained immobile or worked in opposition to movements that, in a coordinated body, they would be assisting. This creates an awareness of what is "right," which works against future immobility or obstruction.

Some restorations of awareness in the body may have to be achieved only once for important functional changes to occur. For example, when a person has gained real awareness of the mobility of the shoulder joints, that single instance of awareness may free those joints to an extent not experienced since childhood, and the newly gained freedom then can guarantee retention of the awareness and of the freedom as well. In such a case it appears that inhibition of capacity was being maintained by a lack of awareness of what is possible—an awareness provided by the exercise.

Some work is done with images in altered states of consciousness and with accelerated mental process (see the previous piece by Jean Houston). Then a minute or two of clock-measured time, which may be subjectively experienced as an hour, can give results equivalent to what might be obtained by an hour of actual physical work.

Repeatedly, as all kinds of movements are performed, awareness is directed to the body and to changes resulting from the various movements. Gradually, this leads to a much more complete body image and an enduring awareness that may be used to prevent, for example, the reaccumulation of patterns of muscular tension as these are dissipated by the psychophysical training.

What may eventually be expected is a lightness, an effectiveness, and an ease of movement; an expansion of awareness and sensory acuity; and a body-mind oriented to, and capable of, a greater range of experience. Other benefits should also be forthcoming, but it is not the purpose here to enumerate them.

What I do wish to suggest is that a psychophysical system of education is preferable in concept, methods, and results to our present physical education system, whose goals, understandings, and methods are both inadequate and damaging—and whose failures are everywhere observable in the debilitated bodies of the young and the old and in the failure to motivate people to preserve health and the capacity to *live*.

Biofeedback: An Exercise in "Self-Control"
by Barbara Brown

Most biomedical discoveries are about bits and pieces of man's mind or body. It is not that these discoveries are not important; they have saved society the sadness of much disease and salvaged injured bodies and damaged minds. Yet, significant as medical progress has been, it has not slaked the nagging feeling, the intuition, of most people that the occasional brilliance and power of man's mind in conquering nature could as well be turned to promoting the well-being of mind and body by action of the mind alone. As sophisticated as society has become, today's robust resurgence of interest in spiritual healing and psychic surgery is graphic testimony of a widespread belief in mind power.

From the beginning of history, mentalists have challenged scientific authority, just as convinced that mind power controls the universe as scientists are that physical order controls man's destiny. Science has always won, for it is far easier to be convincing with demonstrations of physical cause and effect on your side. On its side, mind power has not been systemati-

---

Dr. Barbara Brown, a pioneer researcher in biofeedback, is the author of *New Mind, New Body—Biofeedback: New Directions for the Mind.*

cally corralled nor put to effective use. Mind power has not existed for most scientific authority, even when it fathomed mysteries or became engulfed in momentous ideologic conflicts.

Then suddenly, in the sixties, like a series of underground nuclear explosions, experiments began rumbling throughout the country that presaged perhaps the greatest medical discoveries of all time. In the frantic research activity that has followed, it has become clear that man may, after all, have a mind resource to control his own being, down to the most minute fragments of his physical structure. Including his brain.

The simplest statement of the discovery is revolutionary: Given information about how any one of the internal physiological systems is operating, the ordinary human being can learn to control the activity of that system. It can be heartbeat, blood pressure, gastric acid, brain waves, or bits of muscle tissue; it does not seem to make much difference what function of the body it is, as long as information about how it is behaving is made available. And generally, the more the information, the easier it is to learn to control the body function.

Most people can control what they do with arms and legs, with eye, face, or other muscles, using the kind of body control called voluntary. But until recently, medical science believed and taught that nearly all other body functions, such as blood flow, body temperature, brain waves, or even residual muscle tension itself, were under automatic regulation and beyond voluntary control. Almost without warning this dictum has collapsed. The new research has shown that people can learn to control even these kinds of body function.

The discovery of this ability of mind is abbreviated in the term *biofeedback,* an ideograph that describes the phenomenon of control over internal biological functions occurring when information about a specific function is "fed back" to the person whose biologic activity it is. It is a compound of a technology and a training procedure, using specially designed electronic instruments to detect and monitor physiologic activities (such as heart rate or brain waves). The individual practices to control the action of the monitor by manipulating his mental and internal activities, and the result is a learned, voluntary control over the physiologic functions monitored. It is a technique for extending the capabilities of the mind to control the body—and the mind.

The discovery occurred when researchers began giving information about body activities directly *to* people rather than recording it to be filed away for their own research or medical uses. It is the return of information to the individual that is crucial to the biofeedback process. In Dr. John Basmajian's neuroanatomy laboratory at the Emory University School of Medicine in Atlanta, Georgia, for example, ordinary people are shown oscilloscope tracings of the spontaneous electrical activity of various small groups of their own muscle cells, activity detected by sensors on the skin over a muscle. With almost psychic power, these ordinary people begin to control, selectively, the minute electrical activity of different groups of muscle cells—voluntarily—just as they can voluntarily control the whole muscle when they want to move it. However, now they are activating as few as three muscle *cells* simply by deciding to do so.

Basmajian further taxes our capacity to conceptualize such mind control by demonstrating that the site of control actually occurs in single motoneuron cells in the spinal cord. His subjects (and the subjects of many other investigators) learn to activate these single cells within as short a time as fifteen minutes, sometimes much less. The precision of the control is extraordinary: To activate one cell independently means that other related cells, normally involved in muscle movement, must simultaneously be suppressed. Yet, despite the facility in learning the control, and its complexity and precision, the human

36

mind appears to be at a complete loss to explain how it accomplishes this extraordinary feat. The reports of most people are that they know they *can* do it, but they do not know *how* they do it.

Or, as in the laboratories of Brener and Hothersall, it was discovered that human beings could—unconsciously —learn to control a body function traditionally believed to be automatic: the rate of the beating heart.

Like so many other experimental psychological studies, this one sounds more like a practical joke than research; yet the results are impressive and interesting. Volunteer subjects were asked to make a device produce different pitches of tones "by purely mental means." A red-light signal was a request to make high tones, and a green light was a request to make low tones. With a little practice, the subjects learned to manipulate the tones. Presumably the subjects did not know that they were, in fact, directly wired to the tone-producing device and that it was the amplified electrical energy of their own heartbeats that activated the tones. When the heart accelerated, the tones were high; when the heart slowed, the tones were low. Incredibly, they remained unaware that their own heartbeats turned on the tones and that it was their unconsciously learned control of heart rate that caused the tones to change.

In the brief span of time during which biofeedback has been with us, there have been more reports confirming its validity than there have been for almost any previous biological discovery in an equivalent period of time. Its implications for both theory and application are almost limitless, for when we come right down to it, there is little about the functioning of human beings that does not in some way depend upon the feeding back of biological information to the generator of that information. The excitement that biofeedback has brought is the discovery that man's mind can process and understand even his own cellular information and use it to extend his control of self far beyond that ever before believed possible.

Take the role of biofeedback in tension and anxiety as the simplest example, but one with perhaps the farthest-reaching potential. The majority of emotional problems, and perhaps a good many medical problems as well, stem from the excessive tension and anxiety of today's fast-paced world, and the tensions are directly and immediately manifest as muscle tension.

In medical science the vast therapeutic benefits of relaxation have been known since the early days of this century. Although remarkably successful in many emotional and medical problems, the medical use of relaxation has been limited because it is time-consuming and requires more patience and persistence than most ill patients can summon. This relative impracticability has led therapists to neglect the fact that it is the intimate relationship between muscles and mind that becomes distorted under mental and emotional tension, that somehow this affects other body functions, and that effective relaxation can relieve those emotionally caused illnesses called psychosomatic.

To many relaxation theorists, anxiety (emotional tension) and relaxation are mutually exclusive. Certainly it has been learned, both medically and psychologically, that where there is anxiety, there is muscle tension, and that when muscle tension is relieved, so is anxiety.

Physiologic studies suggest why this may be true. The tension of muscle cells is adjusted by means of a feedback control loop operating between tension sensors in muscle cells and brain areas concerned with effective muscle movement. The control system, operating something like the household thermostat, compares actual tension with what it should be for a given situation and initiates activation of appropriate adjustments. This linear mechanism is ideal for moving muscles and for mobilizing muscles as a first line of defense. The system does not, however, cope well with the way human beings react to social pressures. By social custom physical action is tempered, submerging the defense posture into an unconscious intention to be ready for action, to be alert and tensed. When emotional tension and its muscle-tensing effect are prolonged, the system undergoes adaptation and the control becomes set to higher and higher levels of tolerated muscle tension. It is an insidious accommodation that leads to the muscles becoming set into patterns of tenseness. Its continuous-loop nature feeds upon itself, anxiety tenses the muscles, and the increased tension of muscles keeps the mind apprehensive. But because it is a continuous loop, intervention can be either in the mind or in the muscles. Effective psychotherapy can relieve muscle tension, and effective relaxation procedures can relieve anxiety.

Biofeedback-assisted relaxation is so reasonable that it is surprising it has taken so long to discover. With its ability to amplify a hundredfold, it detects that muscle tension persisting even when the muscles appear at complete rest, the tension built up from social pressures. This residual tension is amplified and converted to a form of electrical energy that can operate meters or any other convenient signal. Because a signal like a meter constantly reads and displays the tension, it can be perceived as it fluctuates over time. Although this is a new form of muscle information, the brain uses it to exert voluntary control over the otherwise imperceptible tension level in the same way that it uses internally sensed information from muscle sensors to move muscles.

In much the same way, symbols of the body's other functions are used to bring them under voluntary control. The diversity of functions—such as peripheral blood flow, blood pressure, heart rate, intestinal contractions and secretions, skin electrical activity, and brain waves—that are responsive to this learning paradigm sharply indicates the intervention of complex mental activity in the automatic regulation of the body.

A strange blindness has prevailed in modern science about the role of the mind in the catalog of human abilities. The failure of the mind sciences to conjecture meaningfully about mind capabilities is easily seen in their indifferent attitude about the way the mind-brain can supervene in what we take to be the automaticity of reflexes. Take blinking and winking, two simple, related, but quite different acts: one automatic, the other learned. Nearly every physiologic system of the body has a similar automatic mode for its fundamental operation, and now biofeedback has shown that each automatic control system can be additionally influenced by higher mental activities. Yet, until this discovery, science had put little thought to what brain activity might occur when ordinary reflexes are controlled mentally, as when blinking is done intentionally and becomes winking. There is little, if any, concrete neurophysiologic knowledge about how volition turns into action.

There are other unacknowledged dimensions of voluntary control. Because intention can select and direct *any* physiologic action, it can be deduced that the decision to intervene actively and specifically in an otherwise automatic biological activity may be a function of mind relatively independent of specific physiologic systems. This possibility is reminiscent of metaphysical thought: If intention—the will—can be mentally evoked and applied to a variety of biological actions with molecular specificity, it is necessary to postulate other mental actions of similar relative independence. The *decision* to do something must be implemented; it needs mechanisms to select the body system and to direct or carry out the intent.

As a matter of fact, the biofeedback phenomenon has already rather startlingly revealed a semi-independent role for sensory information. Bundles of sensory information once believed to play a subsidiary role in directing various physiologic activities can, instead, be mobilized to assume a primary role, as when visual information is used to control muscle tension during biofeedback training or is substituted for visceral information to control heart rate. This unexpected substitution of sensory information is a sophisticated action of the mind-brain and one that begs for experimental clarification by its implications for extending mind abilities.

Until biofeedback and the recognition that higher, complex mental processes could alter automatic functions, the concept of intention, or voluntary control, was considered exclusively in terms of control of muscular activity. Yet, despite a century of research, the decision-making part of brain activity has eluded physiological and anatomical definition. The paucity of information about the purely mental activities of the brain is not generally appreciated by mind scientists. The brain scientist becomes enmeshed in the complexities of neural and biochemical elements, while the experimental psychologist attempts to define mental capabilities largely in terms of behavioral responses to changes in the environment.

So the authorities on the functions of mind have data chiefly for reductionist theories to describe the abilities of the mind, theories circumscribed by the physical nature of the brain and physical responses to physical stimuli. Any experiencer of hallucinogens, or any religious mystic, could give more recognition to the existence of mind and its unique place in nature than could any mind scientist. It is as if laboratory man, no less than primitive man, fears the unknown. Rather than seeking to learn and to use the nonordinary capacities of mind, mind scientists (who are mainly brain scientists) have worked to keep the awesome power of mind within the limits of physical confines.

I do not argue that ultimately the brain scientists may not prove out their theories; what I argue is that they have dogmatized rigid inhibitions for using mind, and

41

these have captured our social standards. We have set limits and norms for intelligence and creativity and outlawed flights of mind. It was less science than a changing social conscience that allowed some minds to see the ability of mind to control itself and its body in experiments that were little different from hundreds of earlier experiments that had discouraged such thoughts.

Through biofeedback, we now know, as perhaps we should have always known, that the mind-body cannot direct the activities of the body unless it has information about what is going on in the environment of the body, its tissues, and its cells. And we should have known, too, that if the mind-brain cannot operate without information from the body, and the body cannot operate without information from the mind-brain, then mind-brain and body are not merely connected, they exist and function as a unit. There are volumes of experiential and medical documentation confirming the inseparability of mind and body; yet, professional therapists, by tradition, by certification, and probably by economic considerations, assume responsibility for only one aspect: mind *or* body. Even with the development of psychiatry, medical science continues to impose a schizophrenic therapy on the problems of illness. The capacity of mind to regulate and heal the body, and itself, has been short-shrifted almost out of existence; problems of mind especially are nearly always first attacked by salving minds with drugs.

The unexpectedness of the biofeedback phenomenon stimulates more philosophic scientific conjecture than does any previous psychophysiologic research. It has taken some time for most researchers to realize that this "new" capacity of mind is most likely an extension of the inherent capability of man, and animals, to exert voluntary control over their own beings. Just how we voluntarily control anything about ourselves is still a mystery, but no matter how the phenomenon is viewed, it proceeds from a sophisticated action of the mind-brain. The fact that learning to control physiologic activities occurs without obvious use of conscious effort and without conscious understanding of how the control is accomplished is a dramatic confirmation of the remarkable capabilities of mind.

It has been, of course, disturbing to find that subjective knowledge of how individuals accomplish control of body functions could rarely be defined in conscious awareness. If the sensation of manipulating distant body activities is so elusive as to escape descriptions that can be communicated, then one is led to conjecture that a nonconscious awareness guides the entire process. And a complicated process it is, one that involves sense perception of abstract information (such as a meter reading) about a physiologic activity, one that organizes, associates, and integrates the information, then disperses correct directions to be transmitted neurally to the organs to change their activity according to a predetermined effective objective.

The nonverbalizable aspects of consciousness are a no-man's land, uncharted and unpartitioned, without physical landmarks or guideposts. The scientist hesitates to enter such a strange land; yet, the obvious facility of the mind to learn control over even the most vital of the body's functions can provide the scientist with physical indices for marking the action of the subconscious mind. To chart this long-hidden expanse of mind is one of the most exciting future uses of biofeedback.

The biofeedback phenomenon also generates new conjecture about the structural capabilities of the body. The rapidity and ease of biofeedback learning is difficult to account for by known theory and literally mandates new insights for study of those internally generated mental abilities that shape what our minds and bodies do. If people can so quickly learn to control events in their bodies that they scarcely knew existed, are they reactivating a lost ability, or are they evolving a new capacity of mind? Either conjecture is provocative. The fact that we, and our animal relatives, do voluntarily control our major life's activities suggests that the control ability has always existed. If it were a new, evolving capacity, chances are it would be manifest as an erratic, fumbling attempt to control the microcosms of our bodies. But if, as in Basmajian's experiments with single cells buried deep in the spinal cord, the human mind can learn full control in a matter of minutes, is it because the ability to control single cells has always existed? If it has always existed, has our reluctance to recognize it been because the idea that mind can alter physical nature has been too overwhelming conceptually to our primitive understanding of the physical order of the universe, or too God-defying, to bring into conscious appreciation? Is it possible that man has suppressed a higher level of mental function, one that regulates every cell of the body?

And will the extraordinary potential of the biofeedback breakthrough be realized, or will the tradition that requires substantive proof of the limits of mind continue to restrain explorations of the endowments of mind claimed by artists, musicians, mathematical geniuses, inventors, mystics, and drug takers?

The sticky point is that our society has accepted as a fact a good bit of scientific theory about the mind, accepting definitions of mind as bounded and limited by the physical nature of the brain. The concept that the mind functions one-to-one with brain processes, a theory for which there is really very little data, should not be accepted as an unwritten limit to the faculties of the mind. Rather, because science is a long way from defining mind, it should be just as valid to explore the mind subjectively as it is to explore it by means of the objective measures currently used that are admittedly inadequate, meager, and often inappropriate.

We should by this time be well aware of the powerful consequences of untracking the mind and breaking its limits by means of drugs, the mystical experience, or the emotional overloading of unorthodox experiential psychological techniques. While scientists themselves avoid recognizing the powerful impact of awareness raising, consciousness expanding, creative explosions that have marked the nonscientific society since the early sixties, there can be no doubt about the revolutions in thought and conscience and consciousness that have occurred. New attitudes have developed about war, about social responsibility, about life values, about the environment. These are powerful changes in mind function, which have, in fact, significantly altered our notions of reality.

And yet, as a member of the scientific community, I watch reports of new research that purport to explore the principle of biofeedback, and I see the security blanket of traditional methodology and concept smothering the vital mechanism of a "new" mind, shaping experimental forays and conclusions to conform to concepts of mind that yet other evidence suggests may be illusory. It is like the Western attitude toward Yogis. Until biofeedback, appropriate scientific experts refused to acknowledge the possibility of control of the physical body by mental disciplines. Now that biofeedback has shown that similar control can be attained through technological aids, the conclusion is drawn that the Yogic process is a biofeedback process and that the biofeedback process is little more than rote learning. That such conclusions are drawn without data is ignored; it seems obvious to these experts that the similarities must exist and, more comfortingly, that the model for explaining human behavior can be preserved intact. And they continue to forget that the model does not explain why and how we select our goals, or what intention and creativity are.

For the immediate, practical applications of biofeedback, it may make little difference how the nature of the phenomenon is viewed, that is, whether one views it as a mechanical learning contingent upon rewards or as a

45

capacity of mind in which complex mental processes can be marshaled by other complex mental processes that give rise to intent and direction. It will make no difference how the effect occurs, for the ability of the mind to exert voluntary control over body functions can be used effectively to relieve a startling number of distressing conditions of body and mind. Biofeedback has been successful in an unbelievable array of problems of health: tension and migraine headaches, cardiac irregularities, high blood pressure, peripheral vascular disease, gastric ulcer, insomnia, epilepsy, asthma, spasticity, learning problems in children, and a host of other troublesome medical and psychological problems in human beings. And along the way it is opening the door to a more holistic approach to therapy.

The future of biofeedback is uncertain only because no one knows the limits of mental control of mind and body. A wide variety of physical and emotional illnesses are certain to be relieved. We should be able to learn how to keep our bodies and minds in states of good health because we now have the means to become aware of their best operating conditions. We have only now begun to explore what all our brain waves mean to human mental activity, and it seems likely that in the future we will be able to control many of the numerous specific brain waves as well as patterns of brain waves that reflect the activities of our minds and states of consciousness. We should be able to become so aware of the best states of mind and body that we can achieve both internal harmony and harmony with the universe.

The Consciousness
Revolution
—— • ——
by John W. White

A consciousness revolution is occurring throughout our culture. We can date it approximately from the beginning of psychedelic-drug research, although its roots go back much farther. In fact, traditions such as philosophy, religion, esoteric psychology, and the humanities have been concerned with it for millennia. But not until recently has consciousness itself become mainstream, and now it is happening everywhere: meditation, psychic phenomena, the don Juan and *Jonathan Livingston Seagull* books, classes in Yoga and mind control, occult practices such as astrology and tarot, psychic plant research, and the use of drugs. Thus, on the farthest frontiers of a host of exotic disciplines, researchers are discovering—or at least claiming with conviction—that consciousness is the primary factor in all experience, the fundamental ground of all knowing, all perception, all states of being.

From all this activity, the dim outlines of a science of consciousness are emerging. Since 1967 it has been called "noetics," a term coined by Dr. Charles Musès,

John W. White is a free-lance writer and teacher. His books include *The Highest State of Consciousness, What Is Meditation?,* and *Frontiers of Consciousness.*

47

mathematical investigator and editor of the now-defunct *Journal for the Study of Consciousness;* he defined it as "the science of the study of consciousness and its alterations." Astronaut Edgar D. Mitchell has popularized the term since he retired from the military; in 1973 he established a research organization—the Institute of Noetic Sciences, now located in Menlo Park, California—to investigate the nature of consciousness and human potential.

Also, 1973 saw the creation of several journals devoted solely to consciousness research. And that year the Smithsonian Institution sponsored a public symposium of brain researchers, psychopharmacologists, psychologists, and biofeedback and dream researchers to discuss their work and its implications for society. Sober publications, such as *Science* and *The New York Times,* reported on the symposium, and consciousness research reached the Establishment.

With that brief introduction, let us look at what consciousness research is doing in some thirteen related frontiers:

ALTERED STATES OF CONSCIOUSNESS (ASCs). This is a catchall term for research on sleep, dreams, trance, and other states of awareness. (See Jean Houston's "Putting the First Man on Earth," page 15, for some uses of ASCs.) A state of consciousness should not be equated with the tool or technique used for inducing or attaining it. Drugs, hypnosis, and meditation can give access to a wide variety of ASCs. (So can reading a good book or contemplating a beautiful day.) Hence there is no such thing as *the* drug, hypnotic, or meditative state. There are only departures from ordinary, waking consciousness—itself most difficult to define—of a transitory or a permanent nature. Some may be "lower" (coma and alcoholic inebriation); some may be "higher" (ecstasy and mystical enlightenment).

BIOFEEDBACK. This field is discussed elsewhere in this

book by Barbara Brown (page 34). Here it is enough to say that although biofeedback is not electronic Yoga (a term derived from some early b/f enthusiasts), its value in helping people to take conscious, voluntary control of body functions cannot be underestimated. The potential of biofeedback is great in many fields—medicine, psychiatry, business, education, athletics, space travel, and psychic research, among others.

Perhaps the most dramatic aspect is brain-wave control. During the sixties the pioneering work of Dr. Joe Kamiya, beginning in Chicago and then moving to the Langley Porter Neuropsychiatric Institute in San Francisco, enabled others, such as Dr. Elmer Green of the Menninger Clinic at Topeka, Kansas, to explore the visual imagery associated with theta brain-wave activity. Green chose this area because theta has interesting parallels with the reverie-like state of consciousness reported by many scientists and intellectuals as the condition preceding the occurrence of their most creative ideas and insights. Green also startled the biofeedback world when he recorded a laboratory subject, Swami Rama of Rishikesh, India, voluntarily producing all four brain waves *simultaneously*—an ability that Rama claims to have learned through Yogic training.

BODY CONSCIOUSNESS. Coincidental with the sexual liberation movement, a wide variety of therapies and growth-awareness techniques, both Eastern and Western, are helping people to "get their heads together" with their bodies and become whole. The Eastern elements include the martial arts (karate, aikido, kung fu, and so on); therapies, such as acupuncture, do-in, and shiatsu; and spiritual disciplines, including t'ai chi, Yoga, and tantra.

The West has contributed to body-mind research with a number of body-corrective systems. These include the body-reformation methods called structural integration (commonly known as Rolfing, after its developer, Ida

Rolf), the Feldenkrais method (originated by Israeli Moshe Feldenkrais), and the Alexander technique (developed by Dr. F. M. Alexander). Bioenergetics, another form of therapy, developed from Wilhelm Reich's study of energy blockages in the body that become muscular "armoring" of emotional wounds.

The newest therapy on the West Coast (where things in this field seem to happen first) is polarity therapy. It was pioneered by Dr. Randolph Stone, who combined Eastern philosophy and healing methods in a system that uses deep massage, pressure on acupuncture points, and Yoga and other disciplines in a holistic manner—that is, considered as a whole.

Better-known therapies are the relaxation techniques called autogenic training and progressive relaxation. Massage, dance, and movement therapy are also widely used for integrating people and opening their consciousnesses to the full life of the body.

Exobiology.   Central to this discipline, which explores the possibility of extraterrestrial life, is the thesis that the building blocks of life exist throughout the universe and that life will develop not only where conditions are suitable but even where they are only less than extremely hostile. Thus, because the sun is a relatively young star, there may be extraterrestrial forms of life considerably older and more advanced than *Homo sapiens*. Where life is, consciousness is. In other words, there may be higher consciousness elsewhere in the universe. Dr. Carl Sagan of Cornell, a prominent planetary astronomer and exobiologist, estimates that there may be more than a million technological civilizations more advanced than Earth's in the Milky Way galaxy alone.

There is an increasing body of literature, especially among ufologists (people who believe in the reality of UFOs—unidentified flying objects), on the theory that UFOs are piloted or controlled by extraterrestrial beings who have visited Earth in the past as well. Erich von

50

Daniken's books and Andrija Puharich's *Uri* are in this genre.

LINGUISTICS. This field has been concerned with the study of mind for a long time. Earlier in this century the revolutionary linguist Benjamin Lee Whorf explored linguistics, going beyond the realm of language proper and into consciousness research. This blazed a new trail, termed "metalinguistics," which has a strong affinity with both general semantics and psycholinguistics.

In the fifties, M.I.T. linguist Noam Chomsky developed his approach to the study of language: transformational grammar. Many linguists and psychologists saw in it a theory of mind underlying the production and the understanding of speech. But initial attempts at M.I.T.'s artificial-intelligence laboratory to use it for programming a computer to understand simple linguistic statements failed.

In 1970, however, a breakthrough was made there, based on two newer theories of language—systemic grammar, the work of British linguist Michael Halliday, and stratificational grammar, developed by Sydney Lamb at Yale. These two closely related analyses of language allowed linguist Terrence Winograd to program a computer to perform some of the functions equivalent to a human being's understanding a language.

Since then, Lamb has extended his work, under the new name "cognitive linguistics," to consider neurophysiological data, and he is now developing a theory of thought processes and mental systems in domains other than language.

MEDITATION RESEARCH. This is another promising frontier. Meditation, perhaps humanity's oldest spiritual discipline, appears in some form in nearly every major religious tradition.

Why should science examine a religious phenomenon? Because of the traditions associated with meditation: the development of unusual self-control over physi-

51

ological functions, the creation of both spontaneous and willed phenonema that do not seem to exist in ordinary states, and the ability to enter unusual states of consciousness in a voluntary manner.

What has the research established? Meditation works on many levels—physiological, psychological, social. It can improve general health and stamina, decrease tension, anxiety, and aggressiveness, and increase self-control and self-knowledge. Drug use and abuse may be curbed, even stopped. Psychotherapy may progress more rapidly than usual. Personal and family relations seem to improve. Meditators claim that the practice changes their lives, and objective research is bearing out to some degree these subjective claims. But the higher consciousness claimed by various spiritual teachers has yet to be defined in scientific terms. Thus, meditation research is still examining ordinary, not extraordinary, consciousness.

METAPSYCHIATRY. This term, coined by Dr. Stanley Dean at the University of Florida Medical School, refers to the interface between psychiatry and psychic-mystic experience. Mysticism, he notes, is defined as a belief in the existence of realities that are (as yet) beyond perceptual or intellectual apprehension but are central to being and accessible to consciousness.

In folk wisdom and literature it has long been recognized that divinity lies next to madness. Consciousness researcher John Lilly (author of *The Center of the Cyclone*) makes this point about the journey to higher consciousness: One goes from orthonoia (a commonly accepted mind state) through paranoia (derangement and rearrangement of the psyche) to metanoia (a Greek word that is usually translated in the Bible as "repentance" but is better understood as "a new state of consciousness"). Supporting this position are British psychiatrist R. D. Laing and Julian Silverman of the Esalen Institute, who feel that psychotic experience can be healthy and growth-producing if it is accepted and handled properly rather than interfered with.

There are others who might be called metapsychiatrists. Norman O. Brown, author of *Life Against Death* and *Love's Body*, stresses that "the disease called man" can get well only by becoming "sicker" in the sense of embracing experiences that have been outlawed and tabooed to disguise what Brown considers the profoundly unhealthy condition called normality. Kascimerz Dabrowsky, who wrote *Growth Through Positive Disintegration*, and A. Reza Arasteh, author of *Final Integration in the Adult Personality*, likewise discuss the psychodynamics of becoming healthy in a sick society.

NEUROSCIENCE. This term covers all orthodox scientific research of the brain and nervous system—which, despite its rapid progress, admittedly falls far short of explaining the mechanisms of consciousness. Some unorthodox researchers hope to get there sooner with some unorthodox answers. For instance, the All-India Institute of Medical Sciences is undertaking an investigation of the work of Gopi Krishna, a Yogi-scientist-philosopher in Srinagar, Kashmir, who proposes the hypothesis that *kundalini*, a Sanskrit term meaning "latent power-reservoir of energy," is both the psychophysical mechanisms by which human evolution proceeds and the subtle bioenergy underlying all mental faculties and psychic-spiritual experiences. The noted German physicist C. F. von Weizsäcker has also taken a serious interest in *kundalini*, though he has not yet conducted any research on the subject.

PARAPHYSICS. This is the study of the physics of paranormal processes—that is, phenomena that resemble physical phenomena but are without recognizable physical cause. Items in this category include psychic phenomena, UFOs, dowsing, and the much-disputed primary perception in plants described in 1966 by polygraph expert Cleve Backster.

Paraphysics occupies a ground midway between physics and metaphysics. Paraphysicists apply the methodology and the data of science to paranormal phenomena but suspect that unknown laws and new forms of energy may be at work. Cleve Backster, for example, maintains that his work with plant communication implies a non-time-consuming form of signal propagation not falling within the electromagnetic spectrum. Acupuncture research, as another example, implies nonphysical energy pathways in the body independent of the nervous system. Some phenomena yield a conventional explanation, however, as Dr. William Tiller of the materials-science department at Stanford University recently demonstrated with the so-called Kirlian photography, in which electromagnetic fields surrounding people and objects are made visible on film.

Tiller is interested in detecting and harnessing psychic (nonphysical) energy. Various traditions throughout history have designated such an energy basic to life, claiming that man is a receptor of cosmic forces. The Chinese called the energy *chi;* the Hindus, *prana* (*kundalini* is a special form of it); the Polynesians, *mana;* the Amerindians, *orenda;* and Christians, *the holy spirit.* In modern times it has been called *orgone* (Wilhelm Reich), *life ether* (Rudolf Steiner), *eloptic energy* (T. G. Hieronymus), and *bioplasma* (Russian psychic researchers).

PSYCHIC RESEARCH.   This field is described in the afterword following this chapter. There is an enormous amount of research being performed around the world, from simple experiments in aura reading, psychometry, and mediumship to elaborate experiments, such as those on Uri Geller's psi talents, reported recently in *Nature* by Stanford Research Institute scientists Dr. Harold Puthoff and Russell Targ. Far too much is happening on this frontier to be reported here. But the significance of psychic research can be summed up this way: It claims to have shown that consciousness can operate beyond the body, out to vast distances (at least as far as the moon!), and possibly independently. If this turns out to be true, it raises new questions about the existence of the soul as a possible vehicle for consciousness after death—and could require a revision of our basic concepts of energy, time, space, mind, and life.

REALITY STUDIES. Early in this century Harvard psychologist William James pointed out that normal waking consciousness is only one state among many and that no account of the universe that disregards the others can be final. "They forbid a premature closing of our accounts with reality," he said.

Since then, consciousness researchers of varying backgrounds and disciplines have claimed that ordinary wakefulness is a mere introduction to the cosmic drama. They have been busily exploring the relation between perception, learning, cultural conditioning, and our understanding of "reality." We now know the human body has built-in filters that select some aspects of a larger spectrum of stimuli and reject others. Likewise, language, cultural assumptions, and received concepts construct blinders in us.

Among those who are investigating the diverse models of reality under which we seem to operate are Carlos Castaneda (author of the don Juan series), Robert Masters and Jean Houston (authors of *Mind Games*), science historian Thomas Kuhn (who wrote *The Structure of Scientific Revolutions*), Joseph Chilton Pearce (who wrote *The Crack in the Cosmic Egg*), and a discarnate (it is claimed) entity named Seth, who communicates through medium Jane Roberts (author of *The Seth Material*).

Throw in the contributions of physics in the form of black holes, antimatter, hyperspace, and tachyons, and Hamlet's words still ring true: "There are more things in heaven and earth, Horatio, than are dreamt of in your philosophy."

THANATOLOGY. The term, from the Greek *thanatos,*

"death," was developed in the sixties when medical researchers turned their attention to the process of dying and death in an effort to understand it and thereby help human beings, especially the bereaved. This remains thanatology's major thrust, but now it has joined with the oldest aspect of psychic research—the question of postmortem survival—to investigate the possibility that death is only an alteration of consciousness en route to another state of existence. One prominent thanatologist, Dr. Elizabeth Kubler-Ross, has declared that her experiences with the dying have convinced her that life after death is real.

TRANSPERSONAL PSYCHOLOGY. This broad term overlaps many of these frontier areas. The fourth and newest psychological school (after psychoanalysis, behaviorism, and humanistic psychology), transpersonal psychology emphasizes the development of a person's fullest potential in all aspects of his sensory, psychic, and spiritual being. Chief among those pioneering this approach in the late sixties were Anthony Sutich and the late Abraham Maslow. Sutich launched and edited the *Journal of Transpersonal Psychology,* the major publication of the Association for Transpersonal Psychology.

In transpersonal psychology it is assumed that a capacity for self-transcendence or self-actualization is present in everyone and that this capacity is biologically rooted and positive—that is, healthy and good. Chief among the concerns of the transpersonal psychologist are cosmic consciousness, ecstasy, peak experiences, universal values, interpersonal encounter, psychotechnologies, spiritual disciplines, spiritual communities, and the sanctification of everyday life—all assumed to be accessible through empirical study and enhancement.

A number of new developments have been derived from transpersonal psychology, including transpersonal medicine and transpersonal education. The latter has already been launched at such universities as the University of Redlands, in California, and Northern Illinois University. And just over the horizon, transpersonal politics?

No one can now predict where the consciousness revolution will take us—but it promises to be an interesting ride.

AFTERWORD:
A Layman's Guide to
the World of PSI
• by John W. White

Nobody can say exactly what "psychic research" is—even psychic researchers themselves can't agree on a definition. But to most people psychic research means the study of happenings, proved or alleged, that cannot be accounted for in terms of the conventional physical sciences. What follows is a brief, neutral report on the shape, aims, and terminology of this field.

The wide (some would say "wild") variety of phenomena being investigated today is either exciting or frightening, depending on one's point of view. Some would include among these phenomena firewalking, UFOs, stigmata, and a host of other occult or esoteric subjects. Others stick to a much narrower area. For example, acupuncture, Kirlian photography, and perception in plants are hot topics for many involved in the field. But to J. B. Rhine, the famous, now-retired Duke University parapsychologist, these phenomena, whether valid or not, are improper subjects for parapsychologists because they are not clearly understood to be psychic—that is, nonphysical—in nature.

Psychic phenomena collectively are called *psi*, after the first letter of the Greek word *psyche*, meaning "soul." Psi

57

can be classified in three major categories: extrasensory perception (ESP); psychokinesis (PK), or mind over matter; and survival phenomena, called *theta* (from the first letter of the Greek word *thanatos,* "death"). Survival phenomena are events presumably influenced by deceased humans or disembodied beings. Theoretically, all these phenomena—which are discussed below—are extrasensorimotor in nature. That is, they do not occur by way of a person's normal sensory or muscle processes.

Psychic research, then, is the field of science that studies the full range of psi, either in the laboratory or in the field. It is millennia old, but can formally be dated from 1882, when the Society of Psychical Research was founded in London to investigate, among other things, the possibility of conscious existence beyond the grave. The American Society for Psychical Research was founded three years later, Harvard psychologist William James being its most prominent member.

In the thirties, Rhine and his co-workers pioneered a new approach to psi that emphasized quantitative, controlled laboratory experiments subject to rigorous statistical analysis. Rhine preferred the term *parapsychology* as a designation for his work. Moreover, although he began his work with interest in the question of life after death, he soon decided that the idea of postmortem survival was beyond the reach of science at that time. So he turned to ESP and PK instead, with his now-famous card-guessing and dice-rolling experiments. Thus, parapsychology is a more narrowly defined, quantitatively oriented field of investigation than psychic research. (The Russian term for parapsychology is *psychoenergetics;* the Czech term is *psychotronics.* However, these terms are more broadly defined.)

The claims made about psychic phenomena can be outlined in the following way—which is tentative, however, and not agreed to by all psychic researchers and parapsychologists:

58

(1)   *Extrasensory perception* (ESP) is a psychic event in which, it is claimed, information is transmitted through channels outside the known sensory channels, either in waking consciousness, trances, or dreams. (The Russian term for ESP is *bioinformation.*) ESP includes:

- Telepathy (Russian term, *biocommunication*)—ESP of another person's mental state or thoughts.
- Clairvoyance (Russian term, *biolocation* or *introscopy*) —ESP of physical objects or events inaccessible to physical vision.
- Precognition (Russian term, *proscopy*)—knowledge of future events that cannot be inferred from present knowledge.
- Retrocognition—knowledge of past events beyond the range of normal knowledge.

When ESP occurs in situations that could be telepathy or clairvoyance or both, it is termed *general extrasensory perception* (GESP). ESP is applied in many specific ways, including psychometry (object reading), radiesthesia (dowsing), and psychic diagnosis. The term *clairsentience* is sometimes used to include clairvoyance, clairaudience, and other expressions of ESP through sensory modalities.

(2)   *Psychokinesis* (PK) (in Russia, *bioenergetics*) is a psychic event in which, according to ESP researchers, something is moved or physically affected without the use of any known force that would allow a conventional explanation and usually without direct contact. PK includes:

- Telekinesis—the movement of stationary objects without the use of any known physical force.
- Teleportation—the movement of objects (called "apports") through other physical objects or over great distances.
- Materialization—an event in which some forms or objects suddenly become visible in solid form.
- Dematerialization—the paranormal disappearance, usually quite rapidly, of an object.

- Levitation (of oneself)—rising into the air by no apparent physical means.
- Psychic healing—the paranormal cure of an illness or disability.
- Psychic surgery—a form of paranormal healing in which diseased tissue is removed from the body without the use of instruments.
- Thoughtography—the production of images on unexposed film by thought alone.
- Out-of-the-body (OOB) projection—the separation of one's center of consciousness from the physical body.
- Apparitions of the living—a visual appearance, suggesting the real presence, of someone distant.

(3) *Survival phenomena (theta)* are events that psychic researchers say are possibly caused by discarnate personalities or entities. *Theta* includes:

- Mediumship—the ability to perceive or communicate with discarnates or to act as a channel through which discarnates communicate.
- Hauntings—paranormal phenomena associated with a certain location and attributed to the activity of discarnate spirits.
- Apparitions of the dead—a visual appearance, suggesting the real presence, of someone no longer living.
- Poltergeists—various paranormal events involving the unexplained movement or breakage of objects, apparently by "noisy spirits."
- Spirit photography—the appearance, on a photographic plate, of images of dead persons not visibly present when the photograph was taken.
- Spirit possession—a state in which a person seems to be under the control in mind and body of another personality, generally thought to be a discarnate (and sometimes nonhuman) spirit.
- Reincarnation—a theory of survival in which some

60

aspect of a deceased person is reborn in another human (but not animal) body.

Since its beginning nearly a century ago, psychic research has greatly expanded its scope, forging strong links with the natural and social sciences: the Parapsychological Association, a professional organization for qualified research personnel, with members around the world, was formally admitted in 1969 to the American Association for the Advancement of Science. This advance did not mean, of course, that all scientists accepted the findings of psychic research. But it did mean that psi could be considered a valid discipline employing strict scientific procedures. In 1973 a survey in the British journal *New Scientist* showed that 67 percent of the 1,500 scientists questioned accepted the reality of ESP or considered it a likely possibility. And here in America in 1974, nearly 100 colleges, universities, and other educational centers were offering courses and study opportunities in psychic research.

Altogether, these facts constitute an extraordinary new interest in psychic research. It would seem that the paranormal is here to stay.

Mind-and-Supermind
in Science Fiction
by Isaac Asimov and Ben Bova

Only in very recent history have people learned to show some pride in the human brain. Throughout the ages, if there was one thing members of our species were sure of, it was that the capacity of their minds to understand or to deal with the world was puny indeed. They were daily faced with the overwhelming powers and puzzles presented by nature, not to mention the riddles of their own lives and deaths. They were at the mercy of every roaring predator. They were visited without notice or prior consultation by flood and storm, drought and plague, earthquake and famine. Under the circumstances, our ancestors would naturally postulate the existence of superhuman intelligences, malevolent at worst and whimsical at best, to account for the diversity of phenomena over which they had no control.

The myths and legends of all peoples are full of gods and demons, awesome in their might, fearful in their

Dr. Isaac Asimov is the author, at last count, of 178 books, of which nearly one-quarter are science fiction.

Ben Bova is a novelist, lecturer, and editor of *Analog* magazine.

mystery. And if there appeared a wizard or magician who was able to control or influence the behavior of demons, then *his* powers were equally fearful, if not more so.

In a word, knowledge itself was dangerous. The sin of Adam and Eve was to eat of the fruit of the tree of knowledge; as punishment, they were driven forth from the garden. Actaeon, accidentally seeing Artemis, is turned into a stag to be torn by his own hounds. Semele sees Zeus in all his glory and is shriveled by the radiance. Lot's wife looks back to witness the work of the Lord and becomes a pillar of salt. Faust, the seeker after knowledge, is led straight to the devil.

With knowledge feared, intelligence suspect, and the mind held in low esteem, not much attention was paid to the workings of our brains until such time as people, organized into civilized societies, could begin to exercise some minimal control over their destinies. Only then could they begin to admire the products of the mind, and even begin to inquire into the nature of its mechanisms. Science was naturally in the forefront of these investigations; and where scientists investigate, science fiction writers will be there to speculate, and to weave their fantasies based on the new feasibilities. Their imaginings in regard to the extensions of mind, brain, and intelligence have gone through many transformations: from the natural mind whose powers are enhanced either through directed evolution or artificial manipulation, to the totally synthetic mind that ultimately expresses itself in robotic or computerlike entities; from mind-on-earth to mind-out-in-the-universe.

The mistrust of intelligence, the view of knowledge as evil, has never left us. Indeed, today's younger generation, coming across this oldest of all suspicions, takes it up and inveighs against modern science as though it had discovered something new.

Nor is science fiction immune to it. Though, simplistically, science fiction would appear to be devoted to the triumphs of science, to the predictions of even greater glories, it is, in actual fact, ambivalent to science. More often than not, attempts to tamper with nature turn out badly. The very first modern science fiction novel, *Frankenstein,* by Mary Shelley (1818), is quite Faustian in its attitude toward knowledge. The anatomy professor, Henry Frankenstein, learns enough about the machinery of life to put together dead organs and imbue them with consciousness, creating the Monster, which eventually kills its creator. Moral: There are some things we are not meant to know!

This trend continued until 1938 when John W. Campbell, Jr., became editor of *Astounding Science Fiction* (now called *Analog*). He insisted that scientists and engineers in fiction be at least recognizable, similar to those in real life (a point the movie and TV industries have yet to reach). Campbell generated stories that pitted intelligence against the universal sea of ignorance and danger. For a quarter of a century, intelligence was hero. With the 1960s, however, pessimism began to gain ground once more. But we are getting ahead of our story.

In 1859, Charles Darwin published his watershed book, *On the Origin of Species.* For the first time it occurred to people that superhuman brains need not have been created *de novo,* but could be developed from ordinary human brains or even from subhuman brains by natural evolutionary processes. The notion that man might become superman entered world literature, even in the works of such titans as Friedrich Nietzsche and George Bernard Shaw.

One interesting example of such future evolution is found in the short story "The Man Who Evolved" by Edmond Hamilton (1931): A scientist (a monomaniac where his specialty was concerned, as so many fictional scientists were in those days) experiments on himself with cosmic rays in order that his evolution might be speeded. (The science is wretched, but never mind.) He evolves first to a glorious specimen of physical and mental excellence, more eager than ever to examine the future stages of evolution. Then he becomes a wizened fellow with a hypertrophied brain, with no emotions but contempt; then a thing nearly all head, anxious to conquer the world (intelligence is dangerous); then nothing but a giant brain far beyond even the dreams of conquest; and finally, a giant lump of undifferentiated protoplasm.

By the 1950s, science fiction writers were beginning to examine the possibilities of evolution from a much stronger scientific background. In Theodore L. Thomas's short story "The Far Look" (1956), two-man teams of astronauts live and work on the moon in thirty-day shifts. The harsh lunar environment forces them to a new understanding and appreciation of human cooperation. Each astronaut returns to Earth with the knowledge that his life is inextricably linked with the lives of all human beings. The astronauts begin to go into new fields of social endeavor, especially politics. Their minds, their outlooks, their attitudes have been irrevocably altered (evolved, in a way) by their lunar experience.

Theodore Sturgeon's *More Than Human* (1953) deals with a collectivistic evolution. A group of five individuals link minds to form a superhuman entity, a group-mind, that is capable of many feats no individual human being can perform. This group-entity is not evil and is, for that very reason, often at the mercy of normal human greed and stupidity.

To dwell solely on evolved intelligence would, of course, be rather unsophisticated. The human brain has tripled in size with almost explosive speed on an evolutionary scale, but that explosion took about a million years, just the same, and that is rather too long for fictional drama. Why not a *manufactured* intelligence beyond that of the human?

An obvious raw material for the purpose is the human

65

brain itself. In the novel *Pebble in the Sky* (1950), Isaac Asimov uses a device that increases the speed of nerve impulses across the synapses joining individual brain cells, and this (in the fevered imagination of the author) makes telepathy possible. Frank Herbert in *Dune* (1963) has his characters use a drug that not only opens their minds to the complete racial memory of their species, but also permits adepts to foresee the future. A particularly skillful treatment of the theme is to be found in "Flowers for Algernon" by Daniel Keyes (1960). This is the story of a retarded adult who is surgically stimulated in such a way as to cause his intelligence slowly to intensify to the genius level. The treatment, however, is temporary and he, as slowly, recedes to what he was before.

New biological capabilities, such as cloning and engram imprinting, have begun to make their mark on science fiction in the 1970s. In Gary Alan Ruse's short story "Nanda" (1972), a Latin American dictator has a supply of cloned bodies stored in deep frozen sleep. The sleeping "copies" of the dictator are imprinted daily with the day's experiences. When the dictator is assassinated, a clone body is revived and immediately takes over for the dead man. Thus the dictatorship is immortal. In Ben Bova's novel *The Multiple Man* (1976), the President of the United States is actually a clone group of seven "brothers," each of them an expert in one field of required presidential lore, such as foreign policy or finance. Thus, a sort of group-mind serves as executive, in secret, while the clone member who has specialized in being the public "face" for the group is supposed to be the only man in the White House.

An older and more common theme in science fiction is that of a *completely* artificial human or superhuman intelligence, with nothing but inert material as the starting point. Actually, the notion of "mechanical humans" or "artificial intelligence" is as old as literature. Originally, such devices were considered of divine or magical origin.

The modern attitude toward mechanical intelligence received its first important launching with the play *R.U.R.* by Karel Čapek (1920). Here we have the picture of a kind of wholesale Frankenstein. The industrialist, Rossum, did not impart life to dead tissue, he manufactured living tissue in a biochemical production line and created untiring, loyal beings to do the work of humans. Each of his creations was a "worker" or, in the Czech language, in which Čapek wrote, a "robot." (R.U.R. stands for Rossum's Universal Robots.) Through an interesting semantic evolution, the word *robot* has now come to mean a mechanical object (usually of metal) that mimics the actions of men and resembles the human form. In modern science fiction parlance, Čapek's biochemical, humanoid creations would be called "androids."

Rossum's intentions were good, as were Frankenstein's, but his robots, like the Monster many times amplified, destroyed not only their creator but the whole human race. This theme was borrowed four decades later by Pierre Boulle to serve as the basis for his novel *Planet of the Apes* (1963). Again we see the danger of a too-intrusive curiosity and the dubious rewards of intelligence.

Čapek set a fashion and throughout the 1920s and '30s robots were dangerous objects that turned on their creators with dismal regularity. This came to an end with Asimov's creation, in 1941, of "positronic robots," rigidly controlled by the "Three Laws of Robotics," which kept robots from ever harming human beings. For the first time, robots were considered machines with built-in safeguards. Sometimes the safeguards worked too well, as in Jack Williamson's "With Folded Hands" (1947), where robots took over *all* human tasks and left the human race with nothing to do. Sometimes the safe-guards are so strong, as in Lester del Rey's "Instinct" (1952) that in the far future, when the human race is extinct and the surviving robots feel bereft of purpose, the machines create a human being whom they can serve and to whom they might abase themselves.

A form of mechanical intelligence that dispenses with the bodily attributes of the robot and keeps only the brain is the computer, a rare instance of a technical advance that did not play a big part in science fiction until after it appeared in real life.

An earlier approach to this sort of thing, in science fiction, pictured the human brain itself, immobilized and kept alive artificially. In Edmond Hamilton's series of novels about Captain Future (which began in 1940), such a brain, encased in metal and bathed in nutrient fluids, played the role of the benevolent scientist.

More subtly, there were human or even animal brains, so immobilized and kept alive in order that they might run complicated machinery, as in "Integration Module" by Daniel B. James (1973) or "The Ship Who Sang" by Anne McCaffrey (1961). Sometimes these brains evolved, through long introspection, into superhuman intelligences who then served as advisers and mentors to normal human beings. The electronic mind, however, carrying arithmetical steps to completion at light-speed, eluded science fiction writers for the most part. It is as though they dismissed the chance of getting drama out of a superb adding machine.

Once the computer appeared, however, there was an instant extrapolation to computers of human and even superhuman intelligence. The computer on the starship *Enterprise* in TV's "Star Trek," for instance, occasionally speaks in a sexy female voice, to the embarrassment of the noble Captain Kirk. The computer named Hal in the Clarke–Kubrick movie *2001: A Space Odyssey* goes very humanly insane and must be dismantled before it kills everyone on the spaceship. On the other hand, in Asimov's "The Last Question" (1956), the history of both humanity and the computer is traced over the next trillion years. Both grow ever more complex, both rise steadily superior to the inanimate universe and, in the end, the final computer becomes God—and starts the whole process over again.

Science fiction writers quickly learned that the interaction between human beings and computers can be the source of high drama. Robert A. Heinlein, in his novel *The Moon is a Harsh Mistress* (1966), and Poul Anderson, in his story "Sam Hall" (1953), both had computer-created personae leading rebellions against repressive political regimes. In "Colossus: The Forbin Project," mammoth computers in the military systems of the United States and Russia join forces and take over the world. In Ben Bova's novel *Escape!* (1970), a young convict tries to outwit the computer that runs his juvenile prison.

And, of course, there can be combinations of man and machine, beginning from either end and working toward the other. There are visions of men who must be mechanized in one fashion or another if they are to withstand the hostile environment of space or of other worlds. An example is "Scanners Live in Vain" by Cordwainer Smith (1950). In *The Dueling Machine* by Bova (1969), men are linked mentally to each other through a computerlike device, for the purpose of satisfying their aggressions by fighting savage duels with each other—completely in their imaginations. Samuel R. Delaney's works have explored many facets of man-machine combinations, most notably in his novel *Nova* (1968).

But there are also visions of robots that lead not in the direction of superhumanity, but, more subtly and movingly, in the direction of humanity. Lester del Rey began the making of his formidable reputation with "Helen O'Loy" (1938), in which a robot resembling a female is made more and more female until we forget she is a robot. More recently, the theme of robot becoming human was dealt with in Asimov's "Bicentennial Man" (1976).

Changing the brain need not be restricted to the advancement of its intellectual powers. A brain can have special powers that the ordinary brain does not have—"wild talents" is the phrase commonly used in science fiction. This, as a story theme, descends from the legendary tales in which some divine or semidivine power grants a chosen human being the fulfillment of a wish, or three wishes. Invariably the lucky recipient chooses badly—for knowledge is dangerous, after all. Thus, Midas of Phrygia asked that everything he touched be turned to gold, which meant he could not eat. He turned his beloved daughter into a small golden statue. He was happier over the prayed-for loss of his wild talent than over having acquired it. In the same way, H. G. Wells's "Man Who Could Work Miracles" (1895)—by wishing—nearly destroyed the earth. In Frank M. Robinson's novel *The Power* (1956), an ordinary man is pursued by a superhuman being who uses wild mental talents for his own evil pleasures. The hero wins only by finding that he, too, has wild talents. The implication is that the hero will prove just as self-serving as his erstwhile enemy was.

Modern science fiction generally accepts wild talents more calmly. They are removed from the divine, shifted into the physiological realm and, in many cases, incorporated into science. In Heinlein's *Magic, Inc.* (1950), as one example, witches and magicians approach the task with the cool analytical attitude of scientists. Randall Garrett's long series of "Lord D'Arcy" stories uses magic in the same way, and for the same diverse purposes that we use science. L. Sprague de Camp and Fletcher Pratt in "The Roaring Trumpet" (1940) and its sequels also attempted to turn magic into a set of natural laws parallel to our own, with people able to travel from one fictional world to another by appropriately adjusting their own concept of mathematics. Indeed, the first sequel to the story was called "The Mathematics of Magic" (1940).

John Campbell, the influential editor of *Astounding/ Analog,* was extremely partial to stories of wild talents and verged perilously close to mysticism in his excitement over telepathy and related subjects. It is therefore strange that perhaps the best of all wild-talent stories did not appear in his magazine. This is "The Demolished Man" by Alfred Bester (1952), in which a murder mystery is played out against the background of a society in which telepathy is an established method of communication. The social consequences of this are artfully drawn, as is the strategy of the criminal who must commit his crime despite the fact that his thoughts can be read.

On Earth there are no brains to compete with the human brain, except for the dubious case of the dolphin. But elsewhere?

The concept of other worlds has been part of literature for at least 2,000 years.

For the most part, extraterrestrial intelligences were, at first, pictured as harmless. They remained on their own worlds until human beings came to discover them as they had earlier discovered the natives of America, Australia, and the Pacific islands. If the aliens came to visit us, they were merely observers, content to comment on our faults. Thus, Voltaire in his *Micromegas* (1752) had a creature from Sirius, eight miles high, together with a smaller being from Saturn, stare in astonishment at human folly.

A new and more dramatic view was ushered in with Wells's *War of the Worlds* (1898). It was written when some astronomers were describing canals on Mars and maintaining that these were the products of a great engineering civilization that was fighting off inevitable desiccation. Wells had his Martians coming to Earth to colonize a more fruitful world.

71

War of the Worlds was the first tale of interplanetary warfare and it opened a new chapter in science fiction. World War I showed the true horror of war once science was applied to destruction, and in the decades that followed, Earth was (science fictionally) invaded from space countless times. Often the invaders were further advanced in science, technology, and even in intelligence than Earthpeople were. Perhaps the most vicious invaders were those in Heinlein's *The Puppet Masters* (1951), sluglike parasites that fastened themselves on a human's back and took over control of his brain and body. Certainly the most devastating are Fred Saberhagen's "Berserkers" (beginning in 1963). In a series of stories featuring these, human explorers and colonists, spreading through interstellar space, meet an implacable foe—lifeless, automated giant warships that are directed by self-contained computer intelligence programmed to wipe out all life, wherever they find it. This is the man-machine struggle carried to the ultimate.

In the end, since it is we human beings who tell the stories, the aliens are usually defeated. This might come about through no direct action by human beings but simply through the force of circumstance, as when the Martian invaders in *War of the Worlds* succumb because they lack immunity to earthly decay bacteria. The defeat could also come through the action of parasites deliberately deployed by human beings, as in L. Sprague de Camp's "Divide and Rule" (1939), or through sheer heroism, as in "Tumithak of the Corridors" by Charles R. Tanner (1932). In making editing decisions, John Campbell was so Earth-centered as to insist that human beings *must* win in the end; he would not allow a human defeat. Unwilling to accept this limitation, Asimov evaded it by dealing with a galaxy that had only a single intelligence, the human being, in his *Foundation Trilogy*, the first portion of which was published in 1942. It was the first time an all-human galaxy was portrayed.

72

There were also attempts to portray extraterrestrial intelligences as friendly, even in some cases forming a brotherhood-of-intelligence with Earthpeople. This was most dramatically the case in Edward E. Smith's *Galactic Patrol* (1937) and its sequels, where intelligent beings of all sorts were combined in support of humane civilization against another combination-of-intelligences that was destructive. In Smith's Manichaean view of the universe, knowledge in itself was not evil, and when used for good would win. Just as in the Judeo-Christian universe, where God is more intelligent than Satan and therefore prevails, so the God-surrogate in Smith's stories is more intelligent than the forces of evil and therefore must prevail.

Smith also pioneered in presenting his extraterrestrials as not necessarily human in form. All too often, an extraterrestrial, except for a few superficial differences (green skin, antennae, two navels), is clearly a primate and usually merely a new species of anthropoid ape. This tendency becomes an understandable necessity in the movies and TV, where, whatever the shape of an extraterrestrial intelligence, it is a human actor who must be converted into that shape. Smith, however, with the greater freedom of the printed word, had intelligent dragons, intelligent featureless cylinders, intelligent gaseous beings. Since then, science fiction writers have branched out in both directions. We have had intelligent astronomical objects in Fred Hoyle's *The Black Cloud* (1958) and intelligent protozoa in James Blish's "Surface Tension" (1952).

About a quarter of a century ago, Arthur C. Clarke commented that human intelligence may itself be but an evolutionary step on the road to machine intelligence: self-aware, fully intelligent computers that can think at the speed of light. In a yet-to-be-published novel, physicist-writer Gregory Benford postulates that biological intelligent species may be inherently short-lived, on the evolutionary timescale of the stars, but that metal and electronic machine intelligences may last for aeons.

Thus it may be that when we actually do find intelligent species among the stars, they will not be remotely human. They may not even be biological entities.

Can we forecast our vision of future-mind? Not very easily. As the Supreme Court follows the election returns, so does science fiction follow the advance of science.

If our biochemists and biophysicists learn details about our brains and, for instance, develop true cures for mental illness, the science fictional view of the future-mind is more apt to foresee and depict a golden age. Even so, the science fiction writer must continue to foresee flaws, threats, and dangers, for he is in the business of tension and drama after all and it is in the streak of tarnish in the golden age that he will find the drama.

PART TWO

— • —

Inside
the Brain

Introduction
•
by Albert Rosenfeld
and Kenneth A. Klivington

This section is devoted to pathbreaking new research on that mere double handful of gray stuff inside our skulls, the human brain. Considering the miracles the brain performs, it certainly doesn't look like much, and it weighs only about three pounds. But they are a mighty three pounds—perhaps the most highly organized three pounds of matter in the known universe.

The brain is the controller, the organizer, the information-processing center of the body. It is the boss. It runs the show. And it *acts* like the boss, freely exercising its privileges and prerogatives. Though it makes up only 2 percent of the body's weight, it hogs 20 percent of the blood supply. Like the leader of a pride of lions, it also "eats" first—that is, it takes its share of nutrients from the blood, no matter what goes elsewhere. In case of malnutrition, it is the last to starve.

To us today it seems obvious that the brain is the seat of mind, thought, and sensation. It has not always

Dr. Kenneth A. Klivington is a program officer concerned with scientific affairs at the Alfred P. Sloan Foundation and has done research in neuroscience at Yale University and the University of California at San Diego.

seemed so. Until very recent times, other organs—such as the heart or even the liver—were considered the seat of mind or of soul. Sometimes the human breath, or even the blood, was believed to contain this vital essence. Aristotle thought the brain's main job was to cool the hot blood as it passed through.

The brain remained largely unknown territory until the nineteenth century. Progress remained slow until the past few decades of this century, during which time there has been a veritable explosion of new knowledge. We are still far from understanding all the brain's mysteries. But scientists have now probed into all regions of the brain, layer by layer, almost cell by cell, and now are down to the molecules *within* the cell.

Neurons, the nerve cells of the brain, are governed, like all other body cells, by the DNA in their nuclei. Though it is still a matter of great controversy (and there is too little evidence to settle the matter), many scientists think that the individual's very cast of mind and mold of thought, as well as all the biological processes of the brain, are written into the genetic code.

One might almost say (and many people do) that we have *two* brains (and this is a distinct and separate concept from the left-brain, right-brain phenomenon that Roger W. Sperry writes about on page 124). There is the conscious, reasoning brain, the analytic intellect, housed in the cerebral cortex, the topmost layer of the brain, and the latest to develop in human evolution. This brain governs the central nervous system via the spinal cord and a network of nerves capable of transmitting electrical impulses throughout the body. And there is the "primitive" brain, the ancient, earliest-evolved brain, deep down, covered over by the intricately wrinkled cortex. This brain, much smaller, governs respiration, pulse rate, blood pressure, and the body's salt balance. It governs the appetites and often the moods: hunger and thirst, cold and heat, sexuality, aggression, and the entire "autonomous" nervous system—including the endocrine system of hormone-producing glands, which communicate biochemically rather than bioelectrically. In this primitive brain may reside much of the "unconscious mind"—the emotional, irrational parts of the mind.

The two brains are, of course, intimately interconnected, often in ways we are not aware of. Every doctor knows that a person's mental outlook can affect his physical well-being and vice versa. And every psychiatrist knows that emotional disturbances on the unconscious level can upset functioning at the conscious level. A conscious awareness of danger or excitement, even "purely" intellectual excitement, can communicate itself to the primitive brain, set hormones loose in the blood, and trigger a whole chain of physiological events.

One thing is clear: if we can understand the brain—the *whole* brain—then we can modify thoughts, feelings, sensations, emotions, attitudes, and many functions we think of as purely bodily in nature. To modify the brain would thus be to modify behavior. The new knowledge indeed suggests that virtually complete control might be exercised through the physical manipulation of the brain, and here the term *physical* is used to include chemical, biological, electrical: the *matter* of the brain, rather than what we customarily think of as the psyche or the spirit.

In fact, many brain investigators believe that matter and mind (or spirit) are one—that when matter is organized with sufficient complexity, it begins to manifest the qualities we associate with mind. It has been shown, for instance, that mental illness or disturbance often is accompanied by changes in the chemistry of the brain, and a now-famous maxim is: "No twisted thought without a twisted molecule."

Using the same metaphor, if we could "untwist" those twisted molecules, we might hope to alleviate or cure many forms of mental illness. If the original disturbance was caused by environmental or social factors, then, of course, physical remedies would serve only as interim tranquilizing agents until the environmental and social factors were dealt with.

What other desirable results might we conceivably gain from intervening in the brain's processes?

Well, each of us would like to think more clearly. We would like to experience our sensations more joyfully, to keep ourselves mentally and physically healthy, to learn and remember better, to "know who we are" with a greater sense of wisdom and maturity, to be more creative. It all depends on our individual goals. Here again, though we might be helped by physical controls, true and long-lasting sanity can be attained, and maintained, only in a congenial human environment and in a sane society.

The prospect of the human brain in control of the human brain does not evoke unanimous enthusiasm. Nor should it. Even matters of individual prerogative are controversial; not everyone agrees, for example, that it's all right for a person to hallucinate in private on LSD. What sets off our real alarm signals, however, is the thought of some individuals (other than benevolent therapists ministering to consenting subjects or patients) controlling the brains of others. In that case, the individual owner of the controlled brain is not necessarily the one whose goals would be served.

Not that brain or mind control is a new idea. Many individual brains have been controlled, to some degree, via drugs or hypnosis. Some nations have developed to a high degree of precision—and have not hesitated to practice—the by now well-known technique of psychological "brainwashing." Moreover, we routinely exercise control, or seek to, over people's minds in many ways—through persuasion, advertising, propaganda, education. Physical control, however, does add a special dimension with its own special dangers and implications.

80

Fortunately, most brain investigators—including those whose work is described in the following pages—are responsible scientists who are aware of the implications of their work. As an added protection, many bioethicists have become specialists in this very area of concern, and they are increasingly listened to. It seems unlikely that our new knowledge of the brain will be applied without careful scrutiny and forethought. Neuroscientists, by and large, when they think about "brain control," do not envision new means for the mass manipulation of behavior, but rather an understanding that will enable free individuals to attain better command of the quality of their own living experience.

A Layman's Guide
to the Brain
by Albert Rosenfeld
and Kenneth A. Klivington

The brain is believed to contain something on the order
of 100 billion cells. Of these, 90 billion are the so-called
glial cells, named from the Greek word for glue. They are
the bricks and mortar, the supporting structure, as well
as the indispensable service organization, of the *real*
brain; the remaining 10 billion cells—the nerve cells, or
neurons—form the "substance" of the thinking-and-
feeling instrument by which we sense our own existence.
When we speak of brain cells, neurons are what we usually mean.

These cells are not evenly distributed throughout the
brain. In some areas they are packed together at a den-
sity of 100 million to the cubic inch. And each neuron
may be connected with as many as *60,000* others, no two
of which are exactly alike.

Every neuron is a highly sophisticated data-process-
ing unit, screening thousands of incoming signals and
deciding how and when to respond. A single neuron
contains millions of RNA molecules—those molecules
that carry the genetic instructions from the DNA and
translate them into protein manufacture. All in all, the
neurons are equipped to turn out 100,000 varieties of

protein. Even with the most advanced computers to assist it, the human brain can hardly grasp its own complexity.

The brain is divided into sections, called lobes, by deep grooves. Each lobe is associated with some specific function, although these divisions are not clearcut. The rearmost lobe, the *occipital* lobe, is associated primarily with seeing. The *temporal* lobe, located directly under the temple, is largely concerned with hearing and also plays a prominent role in memory. The *frontal* lobe is vaguely associated with judgment and other elusive aspects of personality.

The outer surface of the human brain, called the cerebral cortex, is grayish pink and deeply wrinkled. Its consistency is something like that of very thick custard. The covering, or cortex (from the Latin word for "bark"), is only about one-tenth of an inch thick, but it is presumably responsible for man's higher mental capabilities. As creatures with greater mental capacity evolved, their brains became increasingly wrinkled and crumpled in appearance as the ratio of cortex (or surface) to the brain's volume increased, reaching its highest level in man.

The brain and spinal cord make up the *central nervous system* (CNS). The CNS can be divided into essentially three parts, in accord with its three major functions:

(1) INPUT. The outside world can be thought of as *putting* information into the CNS in a constant flow—but the CNS is very selective about the information it accepts; otherwise, we would be inundated with unmanageable quantities of data. The input is, thus, what those cells called *sensory receptors* are designed to accept from the world's output—for example, light for the eye, sound for the ear, temperature variations for the skin—which they then translate into the electrical language of the CNS.

(2) OUTPUT. A segment of the CNS is charged with *putting out* commands, especially to the muscles. In walking, for instance, many muscles have to know exactly how much to move or contract, in which direction, and with what amount of force—and all in precisely timed coordination. This orchestration is the job of the *cerebellum,* which sits atop the medulla and serves as traffic manager for signals headed into and out of the spinal cord. (The elements that govern muscle movement constitute the *motor system.*)

(3) CENTRAL PROCESSING. Most brain cells (neurons) are concerned with interpreting sensory input and deciding what to do in specific situations. This executive process is aided by previous experience stored in the memory. (*Memory,* incidentally, does not seem to be stored in any particular part of the brain, but is, rather, a property shared more or less by all the cells.)

Just as the CNS is an information-processing system, so is the individual brain cell, on a miniature scale. All neurons share certain common properties. The "typical" neuron has three parts essential to its function. The signal-receiving, or *input,* part, often spread like sensitive fingers, is made up of *dendrites.* On the *output* side there is only a single *axon,* a slender fiber that may be quite long. (Some motor-system neurons, for example, extend all the way from the cerebral cortex to the base of the spine.) Between dendrites and axon lies the cell body that contains the nucleus and other life-support machinery of the cell.

What makes neurons special among the body cells is the *excitable membrane* that surrounds them. This membrane contains a molecular pump that expels electrically charged particles from within the cell so that a small voltage normally appears across it. When a neuron is activated, the electrical resistance of a portion of

84

its membrane drops sharply, as if a short circuit had occurred, so the voltage across it suddenly changes. The resultant electric "blip" propagates from one end of the axon to the other. Only the *time between* these neural impulses is variable; the size and duration are fixed for any one neuron. It is possible, using an extremely fine wire inserted into the brain, to record these impulses—impulses of which the language of the brain is composed.

Associated with excitation and inhibition of a neuron are small fluctuations in the voltage across its membrane. The combined effect of these fluctuations in millions of neurons in various regions of the brain is what produces the electroencephalogram, or EEG, the signal—measured in millionths of a volt—that can be picked up by wires on the scalp.

Between the axon of one neuron and either a dendrite, or the cell body itself of the next neuron, is a break in the transmission line. This gap, or *synapse,* deserves special attention because of the peculiar method of getting information from one cell to another. Just as there are many kinds of neurons, so there are many varieties of synapses, but the pattern of action for most of them is simple. When the neural impulse reaches the end of the axon, it causes that cell to squirt a minute amount of a chemical *neurotransmitter* into the synapse. The molecules of the transmitter chemical cause a change in the membrane of the dendrite or cell body on the other side of the synapse—a change that may be either excitatory or inhibitory. Since one neuron may receive stimuli from many thousands of others, the net effect of all the excitatory and inhibitory inputs will determine whether that cell fires or remains silent. This is the decision-making process that is central to the executive role of the brain.

Sensory receptors cover the surface of the body. Each

is specially designed to receive physical or chemical stimuli and consequently initiate an impulse in a neuron connected to it—the first sensory neuron traveling toward the brain. These electrical signals from eyes, ears, skin, nose, or tongue will eventually be interpreted as sight, sound, touch, smell, or taste. The first sensory neuron carries the effects of stimulation either into the spinal cord (if the receptor is on the body surface) or directly into the brain if the receptor lies on the head (the auditory nerve is a bundle of nerve fibers running from ear to brain). Axons of sensory nerve fibers relay their messages to a second set of neurons once they enter the brain or spinal cord.

Cell bodies of the next set of neurons on the transmission line are clustered together in *nuclei* of cells (not to be confused with the *nuclei* within the cells), all of which have similar functions. These nuclei are connected to one another by bundles of axons, many of which are covered with an insulating layer of fatty material called *myelin*. Sensory signals usually pass through several synapses as they travel to higher levels within the brain, one in the spinal cord, one at the base of the brain—the *medulla*—one in the *midbrain*, one in the *thalamus*, the major distribution center for all sensory information, which is located at the very center of the head, and, eventually, arrive at the cerebral cortex. All of the myelinated bundles of nerve fibers constitute the white matter of the brain; the nuclei, including the cerebral cortex, the gray matter.

Neurons are more than simple repeaters of the information they receive. As sensory information passes from nucleus to nucleus in the brain, we find that neurons respond to increasingly abstract aspects of the patterns of sound, light, or whatever stimulus. In the visual system, for example, cells in the retina may respond best to a spot of light of a certain size. At an early relay station in the thalamus, cells also respond to spots, but with sharper boundaries. Further on in the cortex, some cells "see" only strips of light with a specific orientation. Others are still more selective and respond to the length of the slit as well.

Similar principles apply to other sensory systems. The process of passing on information about only certain select aspects of the stimulus and throwing out the rest is *feature extraction*, presumably saving those features of the stimulus that are important for the brain to receive.

Many of the brain's "housekeeping" duties are performed by the *hypothalamus*, a set of small cell clusters (nuclei) collected together on the underside of the brain, below the thalamus. Here are located the "thermostat," which regulates temperature response, and the "appestat," which tells us when we are hungry or thirsty. The hypothalamus also controls the entire endocrine system by controlling the *pituitary*, the so-called master gland, which cannot release any of its hormones until the hypothalamus has first sent out its "releasing factors."

Another set of nuclei related to the hypothalamus forms a loop around the thalamus and interconnects with other nuclei throughout the brain. This loop of nuclei makes up the *limbic system*, which is involved largely with the expression of emotions.

Also much involved in the emotions, especially aggression, is the *amygdala*, which is buried deep in the temporal lobe. Surgical removal of the amygdala can have a quieting effect on even the most aggressive of creatures.

Other parts of the brain have to do with the production and regulation of movement. Chief among these is the *extrapyramidal system*, made up of several nuclei found near the core of the brain.

AFTERWORD:
Psychochemistry
of the Brain
___•___
by Richard Restak

Because chemicals clearly play such an important role in brain function, particularly as neurotransmitters, it is not surprising that many compounds can affect the brain, causing changes in mental state and behavior. Countless drugs have been used, legally and illegally, to stimulate the lethargic, to calm the hyperactive, and to produce "altered states of consciousness." Such drugs as chlorpromazine, a tranquilizer that revolutionized the clinical care of schizophrenics, offer promise for the treatment of mental disease and a better understanding of normal behavior.

Substances that affect mood, thought, or behavior are termed *psychotropic* agents or *psychochemicals.* They include *tranquilizers,* such as Valium; *sedatives,* such as barbiturates; *stimulants,* such as amphetamines ("speed"); and *hallucinogens,* such as LSD ("acid"). Our knowledge of the way these agents work is far from complete, but in some cases we can map out the brain parts involved and make some educated guesses about the processes responsible.

Experiments show that amphetamine interferes with the normal operation of a class of neurotransmitters

---

Neurologist Richard Restak, author of *Premeditated Man,* is currently at work on a series of profiles of contemporary scientists.

called *catecholamines,* of which the most common are *dopamine* and *norepinephrine.* Neurons containing these substances seem to be confined largely to certain well-defined regions of the brain. Amphetamine forces such cells to release their transmitters; in some cases this can explain the drug's effects.

Speak, Memory:
The Riddle of Recall
and Forgetfulness
by Maya Pines

Every day, the forty-nine-year-old man reads the same copy of the *Reader's Digest,* which seems eternally new to him. If you meet him, he appears quite normal—but if you leave the room for fifteen minutes and then return, he thinks he has never seen you before. He cannot recognize his next-door neighbors. His family moved to their present house twenty-two years ago, shortly after he had a brain operation to relieve him of severe epilepsy. As a result of this operation (which was experimental and has never been performed on anyone else in the same way, now that its effects on memory are known), he cannot form new memories. Unlike some victims of amnesia, he remembers his early past very clearly, but every new thing he does, says, sees, or feels disappears from his mind so quickly that his own life since 1953 remains a total blank.

Thousands of old people suffer from mild forms of such impairment, simply as a result of their age. "My mind is like a sieve," complains an eighty-five-year-old woman. "I don't remember anything I read in the

Maya Pines, who is the author of *The Brain Changers,* has contributed numerous articles about science to national magazines.

newspaper—don't know why I read it. But I remember very clearly what happened long ago. . . ." Many other persons have transient, but frightening, lapses of memory after receiving shock treatment for depression.

Memory sometimes fails, but it can also preserve events with extraordinary precision and detail for nearly a century after they have occurred. We still know very little about this precious quality. Nevertheless, we are beginning to control it. Scientists can already improve or destroy the memory of animals with surprising ease. And now, amid much excitement, a new crop of drugs that might help the aged to retain their memories is about to be tested. However, scientists, such as Dr. James McGaugh of the University of California, Irvine, warn that it will take at least a decade before such drugs—if they work—go past the experimental stage.

The past two years have been especially rewarding for memory researchers, whose subject has always been the most difficult and exasperating of all areas of the brain sciences. For a long time progress was slow because it was thought that memory depended entirely on electrical activity—on electrical circuits in various parts of the brain that laid down lasting patterns, or "engrams." Harvard's famed neuropsychologist Karl Lashley spent a lifetime looking for such engrams. Convinced that they must be located somewhere in the cortex, he trained thousands of rats to run mazes and learn other skills, then systematically cut out piece after piece of their cortices, expecting that at some point this would also wipe out the memory of their training. But no matter where he cut, the memory survived. Even when the brain injury was severe enough to make the animal limp or stagger, even when 90 percent of its visual cortex had been removed, the rat still found its way across the maze. Finally, after decades of struggling with the problem of how information is encoded in the brain and how people learn, Lashley came to the tongue-in-cheek conclusion that "learning is just not possible at all."

About a decade ago, researchers began to emphasize the chemical aspect of memory. Whatever memory consisted of, it clearly had to have some chemical component; otherwise, long-term memories would not survive deep-freeze hibernation, electroconvulsive shock, coma, anesthesia, or other conditions that radically disrupt the electrical activity of the brain. A chemical trace would also explain why memories are so widespread—why the engram eluded all who tried to find its specific location in the brain.

The chemical approach led to a series of intriguing experiments in the United States and abroad. At the University of Michigan's Mental Health Research Institute, for example, Dr. Bernard Agranoff, a biochemist, began to inflict memory losses on goldfish. After his treatments, the fish had much in common with the old woman who complained that she could not remember what she had just read in the morning paper. Dr. Agranoff did not cut anything out of the brains of the goldfish, nor did he do any permanent damage to them. He merely injected some puromycin, an antibiotic that blocks the formation of protein, into their skulls immediately after they had learned a new skill, and the skill vanished.

It vanished because, according to current theories, there are several stages of memory—short-term memory, long-term memory, and perhaps some others in between—and moving from one stage to the next requires a chemical step. Unless a new impression is fixed by some chemical process in the brain, it will fade away. The puromycin apparently interfered with this step.

Normally, goldfish that have learned to cross an underwater barrier in their tank whenever a light is flashed (in order to avoid a mild electric shock) will remember this skill for at least one month. In order to make the goldfish forget it, Agranoff had to inject his puromycin immediately after the training session. If he waited as long as one hour, it was too late—the memory had been fixed. He could also administer the injections *before* the training began; in that case, the fish would learn to avoid shocks just as rapidly as any other fish and would even remember it for a short time, but three days later all memory of the training had disappeared. This finding showed that the chemical had no effect on the acquisition of memory but acted on its consolidation, which occurred during the hour immediately following the event.

Entranced by the possibility of wiping out specific memory of something just learned—of a murder, perhaps, or the location of military secrets—in this fashion, a reporter once asked Dr. Agranoff, only half in jest, whether the CIA had been in touch with him about his work. Agranoff smiled and replied, "I forget." His own experiments have been limited to animals, however, and he is quick to point out that puromycin could have lethal effects on man. Almost defensively, he emphasizes that his real goal is to learn how memory deficits occur in the aged and in people with degenerative neurological disease, so as to prevent this loss. "The only way we have to study the fixation process is to disrupt it," he declared.

If the consolidation of memory could be disrupted, could it also be improved? At Irvine, Dr. McGaugh decided to give it a try. Years earlier, he remembered, Karl Lashley had shown that animals would learn new skills more rapidly if they were given stimulants such as strychnine before the training. The results of these experiments were difficult to interpret, however. The drug might simply have made the animals more alert or more eager for the food reward; it did not necessarily affect their memory. To clarify the situation, McGaugh left a group of rats alone during their training and *then* injected the strychnine. He saw at once that the more strychnine he gave them, up to a point, the better they learned. Instead of going to the wrong arm of a maze about twenty-five times before grasping that they had to choose the white alley at every turn, the rats that had received the largest dose of the drug learned after only five or six errors.

These dramatic results were soon duplicated with metrozol, a convulsant drug, and with amphetamine, although these two chemicals had to be injected within fifteen minutes after the training session, while the strychnine could be given as much as an hour later. After trying several different drugs, in graduated doses, at varying times, and with different kinds of learning tasks, McGaugh concluded that he had made his case. "The robust nature of the effect is beyond question," he declared. "The effects are as long-lasting as those of ordinary memory. What we produce is either a quicker or a stronger consolidation of memory, so that whatever is learned is learned better."

The drugs could even bring back memories that appeared to have been suppressed by electroconvulsive shocks. "We can now block and unblock," said McGaugh, a psychobiologist who is currently vice-chancellor of Irvine. "If we produce retrograde amnesia by electroshock, we can undo it with drugs. But all this is time-dependent."

From the point of view of the aged, the most interesting aspect of such experiments was the discovery (by other researchers) that old mice and rats responded to the memory drugs much better than did young animals: their memory improved even when the amphetamine was injected two hours after a training session, for instance, while young rats had to have it within fifteen minutes of their training. Evidently, their memory-fixing process had slowed down. It might then be speeded up and sharpened with drugs.

This finding led to the hope that effective memory drugs might soon be developed to help old people whose memories had begun to fail. But there remained a major hurdle: all the drugs that seemed effective were either addictive (amphetamine) or poisonous (strychnine), or they led to convulsions.

Enter the hero of this story: a Dutch pharmacologist, Dr. David DeWied of the University of Utrecht, who works with substances that the body produces naturally and are thus much safer. His most recent experiments on animals have led to a tremendous feeling of excitement among researchers.

The new substances are natural hormones, such as ACTH, which the body produces in response to stress. Until a few years ago, scientists believed that ACTH acted only as a messenger, going from the pituitary gland at the base of the brain to the adrenal glands atop the kidneys and ordering them to release their steroid hormones. ACTH was not supposed to act directly on the brain. But it now turns out that ACTH has two different functions, and that one of its components—which does not affect the adrenals at all—is clearly related to the fixation of memory. Dr. DeWied narrowed this down to a small chain of four amino acids, $ACTH^{4-7}$, although most researchers are working with a slightly larger component, called $ACTH^{4-10}$. Judging from the results of a recent flurry of research, this chain of chemicals alerts the memory machine to the importance of an event and orders the brain to "print"—to fix the short-term memory so that it can go into permanent storage.

Treating animals or people with this natural chemical would be much like revving up their normal memory mechanisms. It might prevent them from forgetting certain events or skills—a mixed blessing, depending on how it was used.

Doctors who believe that electroconvulsive therapy is the best treatment for severe depression have long wished for some way to reduce the amnesia that follows the shocks. It is not surprising, therefore, that one of the first experimental uses of the newly discovered substance in human beings has been with patients undergoing such treatment. Previous work in the Netherlands had shown that ACTH$^{4-10}$ would prevent a loss of memory in rats that had been given electroconvulsive shocks. Tests are now under way in Sweden and New York to see whether the same will prove true in human beings.

The next step is to try out these chemicals on the aged. According to Dr. Max Fink, a professor of psychiatry at the State University of New York at Stony Brook, who is monitoring American studies of the effects of ACTH$^{4-10}$ on human beings, the first trials with small, single doses of the drug proved inconclusive. But chemists in the Netherlands have now succeeded in making synthetic ACTH$^{4-10}$ that is 1,000 times more potent than the original and has much longer-lasting effects. This new chemical, called ORG 2766, is awaiting FDA approval for a large series of tests about which the scientists are very optimistic.

Eventually doctors may learn to measure the hormone level of people who have lost their memory and then to correct it, if necessary, with pills. What causes senile forgetfulness remains a mystery, but it may well involve the brain's inability to synthesize certain hormones. Even though the amino acids from which the hormones are made can be found in common foodstuffs, an active pituitary or hypothalamus is required to make them— unless they are made available as drugs. Possibly some kinds of mental retardation that involve poor memory might also be relieved to some extent through such drugs. The memory researchers emphasize, however, that these are only speculations at the moment. They have been burned before: a decade ago, for instance, some scientists had high hopes that memory defects could be treated with RNA, but nothing came of their expectations. They do not want to have to write hundreds of letters to distraught relatives explaining that, at present, there is nothing they can do to help the senile or the retarded.

Meanwhile, McGaugh and his associate, Dr. Paul E. Gold, are trying to put various pieces of the puzzle together. They have been wondering how their experiments with strychnine and other stimulants that improved the fixation of memory in rats fit in with present experiments showing that some hormones do just the same thing. Perhaps the stimulants acted by releasing the hormones, they speculate. Or, perhaps neither of these chemicals is actually involved in the process of information storage. The researchers may have stumbled, instead, on the mechanism by which people evaluate whether a recent experience was trivial enough to forget or important enough to store in the memory files. If so, it is a considerable achievement, potentially of enormous importance for the aged. But, on the other hand, it leaves the underlying mystery of memory untouched.

The basic questions are: How does information of any sort get coded in the brain? What does short-term memory actually consist of? How does a memory become permanently fixed? How do memories change with time, as they often do? How do people retrieve any specific memory, out of the welter of a lifetime's experiences? And how do they forget? Neither the scientists who study behavior nor those who work with microscopic particles of brain tissue or chemicals have any answers. Yet these questions are at the heart of everything that makes us human.

In some cases it may be dangerous to remember too well. The Russian psychologist A. R. Luria poignantly described such dangers in his book *The Mind of a Mnemonist.* The man whom he studied, S., never forgot anything. He had no difficulty reproducing any lengthy series of words whatever, wrote Luria, "even fifteen or sixteen years after the session in which he had originally recalled the words." He did not have to "memorize" data, but simply "registered an impression," which he could "read" at a much later date. Luria soon gave up trying to find the limits of his memory—there were none. On first acquaintance, however:

> S. struck one as a disorganized and rather dull-witted person, an impression that was even more marked whenever he had to deal with a story that had been read to him. If the story was read at a fairly rapid pace, S.'s face would register confusion and finally utter bewilderment. "No," he would say. "This is too much. Each word calls up images; they collide with one another, and the result is chaos."

Finally, Luria discovered the terrible flaw that went along with S.'s perfect memory: because he remembered every specific image, he was never able to single out the key points in a situation. Thus, while he could recite long texts, his grasp of their total meaning was not good. After S. began working as a mnemonist, a further problem came to plague him: he could not forget images that he no longer needed. He sometimes gave several performances a night in the same hall, where the long charts of numbers that he had to recall were written on a single blackboard and then erased before the next performance. But in his mind's eye, he still *saw* them in the same place. "When the next performance starts and I walk over to that blackboard, the numbers I have erased are liable to turn up again," S. complained. He even thought of writing things down so that he would forget them, but it did not work. There seemed to be some failure in the metabolism of his short-term memories: whereas old people have difficulty converting any of these into permanent memories, S. was forced to convert them all. Conceivably, he suffered from an excess of the hormones DeWied has been studying.

We've all experienced some form of the amnesia produced by alcohol. Scientists separate such forgetfulness into two types: (1) *fragmentary* amnesia, in which a half hour may be blacked out while the next hour is remembered, and temporarily forgotten events from the "missing" half hour may suddenly be recalled if something reminds the subject of them; and (2) *alcoholic "blackouts,"* total and seemingly permanent, covering a period of hours or days.

The difference is important, for only the blackout is really lost time. In blackouts people are just as crippled —for the time being—as the man who suffered the disastrous brain operation that destroyed his memory. A person who realizes that he has had such a blackout usually feels, at first, "a sense of dread or apprehension," according to Washington University psychiatrist Dr. Donald W. Goodwin and his colleagues. The blackout victim wonders whether he might have harmed or killed someone. He was fully conscious during the whole blackout period and was able to perform complicated acts—traveling long distances, for example, or writing letters or checking into hotels. But no amount of memory jogging will make him recall that he did these things. Apparently, the consolidation process, which turns short-term memories into permanent ones, is seriously disrupted in such cases, and Dr. Goodwin believes that more is involved than just alcohol. There is often a history of head injuries or extreme fatigue, lack of food, or the simultaneous use of drugs.

Fragmentary amnesia, by contrast, is more like a fog —an alcoholic haze—which sometimes lifts, showing that the events have been recorded in the brain and even put into permanent storage, but have somehow been blocked from the conscious mind. Such memories return in much the same way as do memories blocked by electroconvulsive therapy. That is, they come back in a sporadic, spotty fashion. But, according to Dr. Goodwin, these memories remain rather dim and often have an unreal quality, "like a picture out of focus" or like "a remembered dream."

What actually goes on in the brain during both kinds of amnesia remains a mystery.

In the future, we may be able to select either of two alternatives at various times: we may decide to take amnesiac drugs before events so horrible that we want no permanent record of them, or we may seek a heightening of experience through drugs that sharpen our memory for special occasions.

There is also a built-in danger of abuse. Memory drugs, like tranquilizers and behavior-modification therapies, may easily be forced on unwilling subjects. Children with learning problems (caused by poor teaching, perhaps), patients in institutions, soldiers, and other captive populations might be given such drugs indiscriminately. The drugs might even be combined with behavior-modification techniques, to make these "stick" better—to turn some "aversive" experience into a warning that cannot be forgotten. In other cases, people might be forced to take drugs that prevent the consolidation of memory.

As with all the new discoveries about the brain, we are being offered high-powered tools that have direct access to our identity. What we make of them depends on how effectively we plan ahead, what guidelines we set for their use, and whether we keep a close watch on what the brain researchers are doing today.

José Delgado:
Exploring Inner Space
by Richard Restak

It was the German physicist Werner Heisenberg who gave both fame and a name to a standard scientific dilemma: the very act of measuring and observing a phenomenon often has a direct impact that changes the nature of what you are trying to study. If, for instance, you try to get a "fix" on a fast-moving subatomic particle, the very light you shine on it in order to see it deflects the particle from its natural course. The only certain thing about this "uncertainty principle," as Heisenberg called it, is the frustration it engenders. This was surely true for would-be brain researchers until well into the current century. How to probe the structure, or elucidate the workings, of such a delicate, complex, hypersensitive organ without at the same time interfering with that structure and those workings—and without doing unacceptable damage?

A long-standing obstacle to meaningful study of the brain was the absence of any safe, relatively "noninvasive" techniques that would *not* interfere to any substantial degree with the integral functions of the particular brain under study. This lack has fortunately been resolved in recent decades, largely through the use of versatile and sophisticated electrical and chemical probes that make possible the techniques known as ESB (electrical stimulation of the brain) and CSB (chemical stimulation of the brain).

ESB—the more familiar of the two, since it has been in use much longer—is still generally thought of as an experimental technique for manipulating laboratory rats or monkeys in bizarre ways. But it has, in fact, long since gone beyond the experimental phase to become a standard tool for studying both animal and human behavior —and a well-established clinical procedure for treating certain specific disorders. One of the best-known practitioners of this art and science, as well as one of the world's foremost investigators of the brain in general, is Dr. José M. R. Delgado, for twenty years on the faculty of Yale Medical School. Delgado recently returned to Madrid, where he is chairman of the Department of Physiological Sciences at the newly created Autonomous Medical School and also director of research for the National Center Ramon y Cajal. There are, of course, many other scientists working in the same research areas, and Delgado is not in any sense the founding father of the field—as he himself takes pains to emphasize. But no one has exploited these techniques more intensively and intelligently than he, nor innovated these techniques more imaginatively, nor offered more dramatic experimental demonstrations of these methods, nor written more clearly and thoughtfully about them—as, for example, in his book *Physical Control of the Mind*.

I had the opportunity to spend a week recently in Madrid with Delgado and the enthusiastic, international group of neuroscientists who have joined his team. They are engaged in an unprecedented multidisciplinary program designed to accelerate the scientific understanding of the human brain. Though Delgado has become a reluctant celebrity—often misinterpreted, as is customary with public figures—he has remained steadfastly at his work and continues to make major contributions almost routinely. Among the very recent developments that he considers most significant are these three: (1) The transdermal (literally, "across the skin") stimulation of the brain to relieve patients with previously intractable pain; (2) the use of two-way transdermal radio communication with animal brains, paving the way for future long-term brain-to-computer-to-brain communication in human beings; and (3) the demonstration, by CSB techniques, of the actual manufacture of certain important neurochemicals from their constituent elements, radioactively tagged on injection, in the brains of living, healthy monkeys.

And I would add a fourth, which is personally exciting and gratifying to me: Delgado has demonstrated strikingly that monkeys roving freely in the wild—analogous to free people out in the real world—are much *less* susceptible to brain control via ESB than they are when cooped up in laboratories.

All this will be better explained in a moment. But first let us backtrack a bit.

It has been known since the late nineteenth century that tiny electrodes (wires) can be inserted in the brain for purposes of stimulation and recording. A pioneer in this experimentation was the German scientist J. Ewald, who in 1896 drilled into a dog's skull and inserted in the hole a perforated ivory cone. Two days later Ewald slipped a series of electrodes inside the cone and made the first electrical recording of the brain. Later, in 1930, Nobel laureate Walter Hess improved on this concept by placing the electrodes in the skulls of unanesthetized cats. Once in place, the electrodes were connected by long wires to an external power source; the cats were thus free to wander the length of the wires. Although this was an improvement in mobility, it was still far short of ideal. Could methods be established that would do away with the connecting wires altogether, freeing the subjects to move about within their own natural habitat? Was there a way to eliminate the artificial limitations of the laboratory yet retain the integrity of observation?

This challenge has occupied Delgado over the course of a professional lifetime. Now sixty years old and a veteran of more than thirty years of brain research, Delgado is just getting into the full swing of his creative career. "We now have the technology," he affirms, "to study and directly influence the brain in such a way that its normal function is not interfered with. Moreover, our instruments are becoming an extension of the brain itself."

Delgado's interest in brain research goes back to at least 1946, when he first came to Yale as a young doctor who had been awarded a fellowship to study with neurophysiologist John Fulton. On his return trip to Spain, Delgado was confronted with the lack of research funds and tried to solve the problem by working for a while as a ship's doctor in order to collect, during his shore leaves in the tropics, the monkeys he needed for his studies. During one such excursion, he was even called upon to capture an escaped gorilla; within a matter of hours he had tamed the beast sufficiently to promenade it along the ship's deck.

Two years later Delgado returned to Yale and began to establish an international reputation based on his ESB studies of apes and monkeys. In a typical ESB experiment, fine steel electrodes are inserted via a painless procedure into the brain of his subject—usually a monkey—and connected to one of Delgado's own inventions —the "stimoceiver," which is a microminiaturized solid-state radio device that both stimulates the brain by its transmissions and receives responsive signals. The latest model, about the size of a thumbnail, fits neatly beneath the scalp, permitting multichannel radio communication between the subject's brain and a radio receiver-stimulator controlled at a distance by the investigator. In the absence of bulky gadgetry, free movement of the subject is possible in a variety of settings. By sending various radio "commands" to the implanted stimoceiver, Delgado is able to modify the behavior of the animal "implantees."

At Yale, Delgado established colonies of monkeys and gibbons and developed instrumentation for radio stimulation of the brain. Instead of being confined to restraining chairs or individual cages, the animals could be investigated within the relative freedom of a large colony cage in the laboratory. The next step was to study the same animals in complete freedom. In collaboration with Dr. Nathan S. Kline, director of research at Rockland Psychiatric Institute and pioneer in psychopharmacology, he has been directing a fascinating experiment on Hall, a one-and-a-half-acre mini-island off Bermuda, where gibbons with implanted stimoceivers have the unrestricted freedom of the island. "On Hall," as Delgado puts it, "it is the experimenters—the stationary observers—who are in the cages, and the animals who are free."

Almost from the beginning, the gibbons reacted to ESB in strikingly different ways than they had under laboratory circumstances. In an earlier series of experiments Delgado had demonstrated that gibbons could be rendered aggressive to other gibbons in response to radio stimulation of the "central gray," a deeply placed brain-stem tract. This effect was repeatable as often as the stimulus was applied. On Hall, however, the same stimulation did *not* produce aggressive behavior. It resulted, instead, in the animal running around without attacking. If the investigator persisted in applying ESB, the gibbon would finally become aggressive—but the aggression was directed not at his fellow colonists but, rather, at the experimenter himself!

"This should come as no surprise," explains Delgado. "Aggression is obviously not solely a matter of brain stimulation. It depends on the environment as well. Change the environment, and you will necessarily change the behavioral response. This is a very useful thing to remember for those who fear brain stimulation alone as a possible precipitator of violence."

For the past three summers, the gibbons on Hall have been the objects of intensive and systematic observation aimed at describing their behavior in terms of what Delgado describes as "mobility cycles." For forty-five minutes each day, at five-second intervals, the gibbons' activity is observed and stored in a tape-recorder. All of this data, some 10,000 separate pieces of information, are then analyzed by computer. From this mass of data, Delgado hopes to demonstrate in free-roving animals, as he has in caged subjects, cycles of behavior related to rhythmic neurochemical mechanisms.

"The brain has many innate patterns of activity that recur in cycles," Delgado explains. "One obvious rhythm is the one associated with our perception of the passage of time. What is the mechanism for our time sense? Is there a biological clock located somewhere in the brain?" This question is being explored by one of Delgado's teams, headed by Dr. Garcia Austt. Evidence indicates that within the hippocampus, a curved ridge within the brain, there is a way station of the limbic system known to be important in memory formation. Intrinsic brain waves, the *theta* rhythm, fulfill some of the requirements for a "biological clock." "If we can modify the local *theta* rhythm," he says, "we may be well on our way to modifying the perception of time."

Both the Hall Island study and the search for a biological clock typify Delgado's approach to brain research: the use of self-designed, increasingly sophisticated techniques to probe ever more precisely into currently undefined aspects of brain function. To Delgado, the questions asked about the brain can only be as meaningful as the technology available for its exploration. "The appearance of electrical technology represented a revolutionary change in the possibility for study and understanding of the central nervous system. We are now developing the technology to investigate the mechanism of awareness, personality, and, therefore, our own future behavior. The unique qualities of human behavior have their origin within the thinking brain, and the new technology allows us to explore its working neurons."

From Delgado's depth studies has emerged a radical change in our concept of how the brain learns. As far back as Aristotle, learning has been assumed to be dependent upon sensory impressions. The traditional postulate has been: there is nothing in the mind that was not first in the senses. But this assumption no longer holds in the light of Delgado's brain-to-computer-to-brain experiments, first reported in his book. Its central character was a male chimpanzee named Paddy, who had been implanted with electrodes and stimoceivers for the purpose of "teaching" the brain via computer. The neurons of a certain area of his brain, the amygdala, spontaneously produced intermittent bursts of "spikes" (signals), which were transmitted to and identified by a distant computer programmed to respond instantly. Each time that an amygdala burst appeared, a signal was triggered through the computer to stimulate another area of Paddy's brain, the reticular formation, which is known to produce unpleasant sensations. In this way the normally occurring bursts acquired undesirable properties, and after a few hours of experimentation, the brain was unconsciously motivated to suppress the amygdala spikes. A side effect: the normally boisterous chimpanzee became more peaceful. Paddy had "learned" the new behavior pattern altogether from his remote computer-instructor via instant, self-produced ESB.

"This experiment," says Delgado, "shows that it is possible to have direct communication from the brain to a computer and back to the brain without the intervention of any of our usual senses, such as sight or sound. We now have the capacity to feed information to the brain and 'teach' it not to be epileptic or perhaps not to react in certain ways. In addition," Delgado adds, with a broad grin, "we are seeing that the brain is more 'intelligent' than we ever imagined. We can teach it to respond or not to respond in a certain way, according to the signals we feed back to it." Dr. Irving Cooper of New York is now successfully treating epilepsy by employing ESB via surgically implanted devices—though without a computer assist. Dr. Robert Heath of Tulane University had previously treated patients with behavioral disturbances by a technique known as ICSS (intracranial self-stimulation). What he did was supply patients with push-button devices of their own so that they could stimulate their own brains by pressing a button on the portable stimulator. Other investigators have tried similar techniques or variations of them. Do-it-yourself ESB, as it might be termed, was done in only a few patients, and is, of course, not as efficient as a computer hookup might be, nor as quick-reacting.

A frequently recurring objection to such ESB studies and therapy is the fear that the electrodes may be harmful to brain tissues, resulting in a perhaps limited but still significant degree of damage. "Objections to our electrode studies based on their supposed harmful effects on brain tissue are scientifically unjustified," Delgado asserts. "In one experiment we evoked a smiling response in a monkey over 400,000 times without any fatiguing of the response or degeneration of nerve cells, as determined by examination of the monkey's brain after death. It is reasonable to assume that electrodes can be left in the brain for years or even a lifetime without causing any functional defects."

Electrical events are only one aspect of brain function. Neuroscientists now understand that brain activity is not merely electrical but also *electrochemical,* with vastly different chemical reactions occurring in different parts of the brain. Obviously, then, any complete explanation of brain function must utilize techniques for observing, measuring, and modifying the chemistry of selected brain sites.

For this purpose Delgado has developed "chemitrodes" (and "dialytrodes"), tiny, ingenious devices that permit, among other things, the injection and removal of minute but meticulously measured quantities of desired substances at specific locations. As with ESB devices, the dialytrode must be inserted under three-dimensional control, a neurosurgical technique known as stereotaxis. "With the dialytrode," says Delgado, "we have achieved a truly scientific way of looking at the chemistry of the brain. Traditionally, drugs are given orally and circulate through the whole body, bathing all the cells equally, despite the fact that only some of them need the drug. Now we can obviously be more selective, more precise, with consequently greater opportunities to arrive at useful treatments."

Delgado has already been able to treat certain selected patients—as have other brain investigators—by means of his various stimulation techniques. A case in point is Francisco, a thirty-year-old telephone operator. A serious automobile accident left Francisco's arm paralyzed because of a shearing of his brachial plexus, a network of nerves supplying power to his left arm. Over the next several months, he began to experience pain that rose to intolerable levels. Finally, even high doses of narcotics failed to bring any relief. With neurosurgery accepted as a last resort, Delgado proposed the insertion of his subcutaneous stimulator with four electrodes placed in two brain sites that prior experimentation in animals had shown to inhibit pain. After a period of study, Delgado's team located a cerebral point that, on stimulation, gave long-lasting relief from the pain, as well as the improvement of the depression Francisco had meanwhile developed. Intermittent stimulation was then directed over a period of several months solely to this one area.

Now, three years later, Francisco is back at work and remains free of pain. He is loath to have the transdermal stimulator removed—though he has not required further stimulation, and Delgado doubts that he will ever need it again.

Apart from pain relief, other potential medical applications of the ongoing research are in manic-depressive psychosis, epilepsy, and certain forms of episodic violent behavior that are postulated to be rooted in brain damage or disorder.

In addition, recent neurochemical research in Delgado's laboratory has demonstrated quantitative differences in the tendency of the brain cells of certain animals to "bind" addicting drugs—to hang on to them chemically—depending on whether the animals are raised in isolation or in groups. The "socially isolated" animal binds far more of the addictive chemicals, while at the same time it exhibits a lessened ability to relate to other animals and a tendency toward aggressive behavior. Dr. Francis Defeudis, the project's young director, has cautiously suggested that such studies may play an important role in unraveling the neurochemistry of drug addiction, with its accompanying social isolation and withdrawal.

To Delgado, the isolation experiments provide a perfect case in point for one of his key concepts—that the brain is a dynamic organ exquisitely responsive to the environment. If he is correct, such studies may ultimately do away with our traditional convention of separating environmental influences from genetic or biochemical ones. "We have demonstrated at the molecular level," he says, "that an environmental variant can actually change the makeup of the clinical reactivity of the brain cell."

The idea of the brain as changeable and therefore at

least partially modifiable has obvious social implications. Brain research, to remain relevant, cannot remain a detached scientific enterprise. It must—rather inevitably— begin, in Delgado's view, to touch on a host of social questions, such as nutrition, education, pollution. As one simple instance, nutritional deficiency in early infancy has been shown to cause irreversible stunting of brain growth, even if nutrition is improved at a later date. This cannot simply be set down as a "cold fact" of brain research; rather, it poses a social and moral challenge: how to guarantee adequate nutrition for every human being during the critical first few months of life.

"There seem to exist critical periods when the brain can be decisively influenced by environmental factors as diverse as the adequacy of the diet or the permissiveness of the schools," says Delgado. "One of our goals is to discover through research how our brains are 'molded,' how and why they respond as they do in different environments."

Awareness of the delicate interplay between the brain and the environment makes possible, Delgado believes, a new type of person—the "psychocivilized person." The "psychocivilized man or woman realizes that thoughts and personalities are dependent on culture and education (sensory inputs) *plus* the organization of the brain. Each person is in the middle of a feedback between emotions and feelings, on the one hand, and electrical, mechanical, and anatomical phenomena on the other. We now have the capacity to plan our future destiny by combining an awareness of our culture with an increasing knowledge of the supporting neurological mechanisms that define the limits of our behavior. Because our brains, as well as our cultures, can be modified, we now have the unique capacity to direct our own evolution. Instead of 'know thyself' we might be more appropriately encouraged to 'create thyself.' "

111

Brain Damage:
A Window on the Mind
by Howard Gardner

Over the past decades our understanding of brain chemistry, of neural circuitry, of sensory and motor processes, has so increased as to render obsolete the medical textbooks of an earlier generation. But how much have these lines of neurological investigation—usually conducted with "lower" animals and dependent upon microscopic preparations—revealed about the functioning of the human mind? Can we draw from studies at the cellular level insights about those intellectual, emotional, and social capacities of pivotal importance within human society? In truth, it must be said: the gap between most work in the brain sciences and the elucidation of our own "higher functions" remains enormous.

Accumulating over the past century, however, has been an unexpected but highly revealing set of insights, one that illuminates precisely those functions central in human intellectual activity. From the careful study of normal individuals whose brains have been injured, we receive penetrating glimpses into the na-

Howard Gardner conducts research on the symbol-using skills of normal children and brain-damaged adults. He is the author of *The Shattered Mind: The Person After Brain Damage.*

112

ture of such cerebral activities as reading, writing, speaking, drawing, doing mathematics, and making music. We can uncover the links—and the distances—between such activities. And we can gain fertile clues about those enigmas that have long intrigued both philosophers and laymen. What is the nature of memory? Can one think without language? Are all art forms cut from a single cloth?

An uncomfortably large number of circumstances can injure the adult brain, but by far the most common and —as it happens—the most revealing is the cerebral vascular accident, or stroke. Each year, in this country alone, approximately 300,000 individuals suffer a stroke when blood vessels leading to the brain are occluded by deposits of fat, a clot lodges in an artery, or an artery bursts. These events threaten the loss of the two elements upon which the brain is crucially dependent: oxygen and glucose. Deprived of these precious substances for more than a few minutes and having no reservoirs upon which to draw, brain tissue is damaged or destroyed. And, once destroyed, it cannot be regenerated. Instead, one may await an unpalatable set of failures in those functions controlled by the brain cells: loss of motor and sensory capacities, failure of "high-level cognitive functions," and, perhaps, coma and death.

In the most fortunate cases, injury to the brain caused by a stroke may be so slight that it remains undetected; on other occasions, death or total disability occurs. But a sizable number of strokes each year prove to be of intermediate severity—insufficient to kill, yet virulent enough to affect permanently the individual's mental functioning. By what they can (and cannot) do, these unfortunate victims yield invaluable information to the neurologists, psychologists, and other scientists involved in the study of the brain.

Were the destruction wrought by a stroke, tumor, or head trauma completely general, so that all mental abili-

113

ties were reduced by an equivalent proportion, little knowledge could be gained about the nature and organization of intellectual skills. (The victim would simply be a "dulled" normal individual; any insights gained from studying him might as readily be procured from the investigation of other normal individuals.) In fact, however, brain damage is highly selective. The victim may lose some abilities completely, while others remain wholly or virtually unaffected. An individual with a lesion in his left hemisphere may be completely unable to speak, while remaining able to draw or to hum with skill. An individual with a lesion in his right hemisphere may be unable to dress himself properly and may lose his way in the hospital, while he can read and speak just as before.

As a result of these somewhat surprising circumstances, the brain-damaged patient constitutes a unique experiment in nature. What could never be done experimentally occurs daily as a result of inexorable fate.

As a neuropsychological researcher at the Aphasia Research Center of the Boston Veterans Administration Hospital, I have come to know several hundred victims of brain damage. Most of our patients are aphasic: their language abilities have been disrupted as a result of damage to the brain, such injury implicating their left cerebral cortex in nearly all cases. About one-third of our patients suffer from other kinds of brain injury in other sites, which, while sparing their language functions, vitiate other abilities. And so I have had the instructive opportunity of comparing the functioning of two kinds of patients—those whose language is impaired but who have retained other abilities, and those who, while losing other capacities, retain the abilities to express themselves verbally and to understand spoken language. In what follows, then, I shall sketch some of the insights that other researchers and I have obtained from studying various brain injuries that may befall the normal adult.

114

One of the first lessons gleaned from work with brain-damaged patients is that commonsense notions of the relationships among abilities may be invalid. Take, for example, the set of symptoms encountered in a bizarre but not infrequent condition called *pure alexia without agraphia*. Patients afflicted with this disorder are unable to read text (they are alexic) yet remain able to write (they are not agraphic). One's immediate thought is that they must be in some sense blind; but in fact the patients can copy or trace out the very letters and words that they fail to read. To complicate the matter even further, the same patients often are able to read numbers. They may even read "DIX" as "509," while proving incapable of reading it as "diks." They are able to name objects but are frequently unable to name samples of colors shown to them.

On its own this syndrome confounds a raft of intuitions about how the mind works. Reading can be separated from writing; verbal symbols differ from numerical symbols; objects are named in a way different from colors. No one completely understands pure alexia, but the major facts of the syndrome described above have been repeatedly described and are widely accepted. Some researchers hold that the individual's visual powers and his verbal-language capacities are reasonably intact but that the connections between them have been disrupted. As a result, purely visual configurations—like letters or colors—cannot be named (or read). But those visual configurations that arouse sensory or tactile associations (like objects or numbers) can be satisfactorily processed. Evidently, such findings not only undermine common sense; they also challenge the researcher to devise a model of mind that can account for this bizarre blend of abilities and disabilities. And they provide intriguing clues about why some normal individuals can master arithmetic before they can read or why others can more easily remember the names of rare objects than rare colors.

Pure alexia demonstrates that symbols that might have been thought similar (numbers and words) are processed in different ways by the brain. Other syndromes demonstrate precisely the reverse situation; skills usually thought independent of one another in fact turn out to be closely related. In a condition that accompanies injury to the parietal and occipital lobes of the left hemisphere, patients can understand single words and declarative sentences but fail to decode utterances that employ prepositional phrases like "on top of" or "next to," possessive constructions ("my brother's wife"), or the passive voice ("the lion was killed by the tiger"). Further investigations with these patients reveal difficulties in carrying out mathematical operations and in analyzing a spatial array. These disabilities co-occur with sufficient regularity to suggest that the same underlying "mental operations" may be drawn upon in understanding certain linguistic structures, in performing arithmetic, and in comprehending a spatial layout. And so, in this instance, the modeler of mental processes is challenged to unite skills that, on intuitive grounds, may appear quite unrelated. By the same token, the schoolteacher receives an impetus to use linguistic examples to aid mathematical understanding or to draw upon mathematical exercises in explicating the principles of grammar.

In most cases the deficits exhibited by brain-damaged patients are only too apparent, to the victim as well as to those who know him. Sometimes, however, a victim may be completely unaware of his deficits, and they may even escape the casual observer as well. An instructive example of this is Korsakoff's disease, a syndrome that results from damage to the midbrain and is often the pathetic climax of many years of alcoholism.

The Korsakoff patient exhibits no evident physical disabilities. He may perform at an average or above-average level on an intelligence test. He can solve a variety of problems posed to him; he can converse in an intelligent manner for hours. And yet, once his deficit has been revealed, it becomes painfully obvious. For a victim of Korsakoff's disease cannot remember anything that is told to him or anything that has happened to him since the onset of his disease.*

Few medical demonstrations are as powerful (and memorable) as that of Korsakoff's disease: one tells an apparently normal patient one's name, engages him in distracting conversation for a few moments, and then hears the patient not only claim ignorance of one's name but also deny that it has ever been told to him. Yet, if all memory were of a single piece, the mechanisms underlying this process would not be illuminated by Korsakoff's disease.

In fact, however, the Korsakoff patient *is* able to learn things, providing only that one does not accept his testimony concerning what he knows. For instance, one can teach such a patient to play a new piece on the piano; the next day he will deny ever having learned the piece, but, once given the opening bars, he (or his fingers) will play the piece perfectly. One can teach a Korsakoff patient a complex new motor skill—say, solving a maze or copying an intricate pattern; once again, despite his sincere protestations of ignorance, the patient (or his hands) will reveal mastery of this new skill. And, most surprisingly of all, one can even teach such a patient a new line of verse, a nonsense slogan, or a series of answers to questions.

Such findings document at least two forms of memory. Given sufficient drill, the brain of the Korsakoff patient can learn new patterns—motor, musical, even verbal—and can spew these patterns back under appropriate circumstances. But the Korsakoff patient has

---

*Note the remarkable similarity between Korsakoff symptoms and those displayed by the victim of an entirely different kind of injury—the case that opens Maya Pines's article on page 90.

largely lost the ability to learn something new—particularly if it is verbal. And he is completely incapable of knowing what he has learned or of drawing upon such new skills in the voluntary way available to normal individuals.

The Korsakoff patient, finally, illuminates some of the quirks of our own mnemonic capacities: we can now better understand why we may be able to repeat a game, a motor activity, or a prayer that apparently had been forgotten; why a line of verse may be more effortlessly retrieved when its meaning is ignored and its syllabic sequence is allowed to unfold without interruption; why a forgotten town becomes instantly familiar once we return to its environs; or why we can sometimes parrot back a recently heard phrase whose meaning has totally eluded us.

Study of the brain-damaged individual not only can illuminate the ordinary processes of ordinary individuals; it can also help to unravel highly developed skills possessed by talented individuals. Among the individuals who have proved extremely difficult to study under ordinary conditions are artists; such creative persons are few, are often unsympathetic to empirical investigators, and usually possess skills of such fluency that they defy dissection and analysis. Here, again, the accidents of brain damage offer a unique investigative opportunity.

Only on rare occasions has an artistically knowledgeable neurologist encountered an accomplished artist whose brain has been damaged. But from such rare happenings considerable insight has been gained into the operation of the artistic mind. Typically, painters can continue to create significant works after their language powers have been seriously disturbed; indeed, more than one researcher has claimed that visual artistry actually improves as a result of aphasia. But, interestingly enough, painters with right-hemisphere disease—whose language has remained unaffected—often exhibit bizarre

118

patterns in the paintings: they may neglect the left side of the canvas, they may distort the external form of objects, or they may portray emotionally bizarre or even repulsive subject matter. Apparently, painting and linguistic capacities can exist independently of each other.

On the other hand, the relationship between linguistic and musical skills seems more complex. Some aphasic musicians prove able to compose or perform; some (among them the composer Maurice Ravel) have lost the ability to create musically even though their critical powers seem to be intact; still other musicians have been completely disabled by aphasia.

The striking individual differences found among brain-damaged musicians suggests that musical capacities may be organized in idiosyncratic ways across individuals. Perhaps most individuals learn in rather similar ways to speak and to draw, but the organization of music in the brain may differ dramatically depending on whether one has learned an instrument, what instrument one favors, whether one plays by ear, the extent to which one sings, and so on. No wonder that the preparation of musical exercises suitable for all students poses enormous challenges to even the most gifted and enterprising music teacher!

Of the diverse conundrums that populate the area of human neuropsychology, none is more persistent and more endlessly fascinating than the relationship between language and thought. Opinions on this issue vary enormously. Some investigators (for example, those influenced by American linguist Benjamin Lee Whorf) view all thought processes as shaped by language and consider aphasia the death of cognition. Other researchers (for instance, those influenced by the Swiss psychologist Jean Piaget) see language and thought as separate streams; they believe that thought can proceed in a virtually unimpaired manner despite a pronounced aphasia.

Dozens of studies inspired by this vexing question reveal quite clearly the inadequacy of both extreme positions. Unquestionably, certain cognitive and intellectual abilities depend quite heavily on linguistic intactness: the ability to reason about abstract issues, the capacity to solve scientific problems, and, in most cases, skill at mathematics. (Just try to think about a comparison between Socialism and Communism without resorting to words.) However, an equally impressive list details reasoning powers that may be well preserved despite a severe aphasia: the ability to solve spatial problems, sensitivity to fine differences in patterns or configurations, and alertness to the emotional contours of a situation. (Just try to describe a spiral staircase using only words.) And, though this area has not been much studied, it seems probable that an individual's sense of himself is not noticeably affected by linguistic impairment—even as "the self" can be decimated while linguistic powers remain completely unaffected.

With every passing year new neuropsychological laboratories are opened; virtually every issue of the leading journals documents fascinating new cases or pivotal experimental discoveries. Our knowledge of the skills detailed above, as well as many others not alluded to here, is certain to increase and to change. And yet it is already possible, on the basis of well-documented findings, to posit reasonably convincing models of human mental processes, particularly in the area of language. Moreover, it should be possible within the next decade to begin integrating what is known about relatively discrete cognitive functions—such as reading, memory, or visual recognition—with insights concerning such subtle and elusive areas as the individual's emotional life, his preferences and fears, his relationships with other people, and, most intriguing of all, his consciousness of his own experiences and of the world about him.

Understanding the brain-damaged individual, and extrapolating to the normal person, is a worthwhile scientific endeavor in its own right. I do not at all wish to detract from it. However, work with the victims of brain damage provides both an opportunity and a challenge to aid these often hapless individuals. It is therefore encouraging to report that in the area of aphasia the increased understanding obtained from neuropsychological investigation has suggested some promising avenues of rehabilitation.

Once it had been established that skills in musical and visual tasks could be at least partially dissociated from linguistic skills, the possibility arose that such spared capacities might be marshaled to aid individuals in communicating with other persons. At our own unit, novel forms of aphasia therapy have been designed for use with patients who have not benefited from traditional language therapy. The most successful of these new therapies, devised by Martin Albert, Nancy Helm, and Robert Sparks, involves the use of singing (or melodic intonation) in order to aid the patient who is unable to express himself orally. A still-experimental therapy, which I have developed in association with Edgar Zurif and several other investigators, involves the ordering of visual symbols drawn on index cards. Patients learn to associate these symbols with objects and actions in the world and then communicate their wishes and thoughts by manipulating the cards. Still other therapies, designed with the aphasic patient's strengths and limitations in mind, draw on sign language and on manipulation of an artificial speech synthesizer. It is still too early to pass final judgment on the efficacy of these therapies, but they at least offer hope that those areas of the brain that have been spared may to some extent be placed in the service of apparently destroyed functions.

Because the patient ordinarily studied by neuropsychologists was once normal, those parts of his brain that still function are presumed to reflect the way in which

121

mental capacities are typically organized in the intact individual. In this respect he differs from the young child, whose brain is much less differentiated into specific zones and, at the same time, much more flexible. The adult with even a relatively small lesion may suffer permanent damage of major skills; the toddler can lose as much as half of his brain (via the removal of a hemisphere) and yet remain able to function quite effectively in intellectual matters, presumably because spared areas "take over" functions.

Despite these telling differences in brain organization and potential, knowledge about children's learning abilities and disabilities can be obtained from a study of the brain-damaged adult. In my view, the kinds of brain injuries that befall adults often seem to reveal conditions found, perhaps in somewhat less clear-cut form, in schoolchildren with learning disabilities. For instance, individuals with acquired alexias (or reading disorders) often resemble children with dyslexia (otherwise-competent children exhibiting special difficulties in reading). Similarly, adult patients with selective disorders in calculation often resemble children who experience special difficulties in learning arithmetic. (Selective sparing may also prove illuminating: patients who can decode written symbols or who can repeat language without understanding resemble certain retarded, autistic, or "hyperlexic" children.)

These clinical findings suggest that some children may be born with neurological abnormalities that yield the behavioral pattern found in certain normal adults whose brains have been injured. The rehabilitative clue here arises from the fact that the brain-damaged adult could once perform the now-disrupted function. Should one succeed in devising a way to "reactivate" this skill, using a channel that is as yet unimpaired, one might accomplish two goals. Even while aiding the adult in recovering an ability of importance, one has developed methods that may facilitate the acquisition of these same skills by the learning-disabled child. For one has developed an alternative-training regime that, while unnecessary for the completely normal child, may prove highly serviceable for the child with a slightly atypical brain.

Returning to our original example of pure alexia without agraphia, one finds further applications of this procedure. Studies have documented that, if given three-dimensional letters to touch, alexic patients can read with greater skill. And, more intriguingly, studies of alexic patients in the Orient have revealed that they may be able to read ideographic characters while they fail to read phonetic characters. Just these insights have recently been drawn upon in the education of American children with selective disabilities in reading. Thus, Paul Rozin and his colleagues at the University of Pennsylvania have developed an ideographic system effective with inner-city dyslexic children. And Jay Isgur, working in Pensacola, Florida, with learning-disabled youngsters, has reported marked success in a program that builds upon the use of three-dimensional, "objectlike" letters.

Whether such rehabilitative measures prove to be potent prosthetics, or of only marginal assistance, remains to be determined. Once destroyed, brain tissue is forever beyond repair, and the loss of this substance almost invariably involves serious cost. Yet, given that some brain damage is inevitable, and that transplants of neural protoplasm will not soon be with us, efforts to assist the injured child or adult must certainly be encouraged. And, indeed, such efforts constitute one of the most rewarding portions of research on brain damage. Even as insights into our own minds, and into mental processes generally, have been coming forth rapidly, it has proved possible to apply what has been learned to those individuals who, willingly if inadvertently, have contributed to our understanding.

123

Left-Brain, Right-Brain

by Roger W. Sperry

At the upper levels of the brain is a thick bundle of transverse fibers called the *corpus callosum,* the largest fiber system in the brain, interconnecting the brain's two large cerebral hemispheres, now commonly known as left-brain and right-brain.

A series of operations to remove the corpus callosum was performed in the late thirties and early forties in order to relieve the seizures of persons afflicted with severe epilepsy—the theory being that the corpus callosum transmitted the brain waves that caused the seizures. The operation proved effective for selected severe cases in minimizing seizures or in stopping them altogether, but the most remarkable effect of this drastic operation was the seeming *lack* of effect on the patient's behavior and personality.

Extensive follow-up studies failed to disclose any definite neurological or psychological symptoms or deficits left by the surgery. That was generally the case, as well, in occasional individuals born without a corpus cal-

Dr. Roger W. Sperry is Hixon Professor of Psychobiology at California Institute of Technology. This article is an edited adaptation of a speech Dr. Sperry gave upon receiving the twenty-ninth annual Passano Foundation Award.

losum. As late as the early fifties, the function of the corpus callosum—estimated to contain over 200 million fiber elements—was still an enigma.

This fact prompted my colleagues and me to undertake a series of laboratory studies on surgical sections of the corpus callosum of cats and monkeys. It soon became evident that the surgically disconnected halves of the brain have their own private sensations, percepts, and learning experiences—all cut off from the awareness of the partner hemisphere. We also learned that each brain half stored its own separate chain of memories, which were inaccessible to the other hemisphere.

The split-brained animal, having learned a task with one hemisphere, would have to relearn it all over again from the beginning when it was obliged to use its other hemisphere. Further, the two hemispheres could be trained concurrently to learn mutually contradictory solutions to a task—with no apparent mental conflict. It was as if each hemisphere was a mind of its own.

This finding, however, still did not tell us much about the left-brain, right-brain differences in people, because it turns out that human beings are the only mammals whose left and right brains are specialized for quite different *functions.* This phenomenon is correlated with the power of speech and the related talents that separate us so distinctly from all other animals.

Our first opportunity to study a human split brain came in 1962, when a callosum-cutting operation was performed by Philip Vogel and Joseph Bogen of the White Memorial Medical Center in Los Angeles. The patient was a forty-eight-year-old war veteran whose brain had been severely damaged by bomb fragments. The injury afflicted him with terrible convulsive seizures, which continued to worsen in spite of all treatment. Upon recovery from the surgery, he was free of the seizures and seemed quite normal in his everyday behavior;

125

in fact, he even showed a much improved sense of well-being. But his surface normality seemed, after more analytic testing, to overlie some startling changes in his inner mental makeup—a suspicion we were to confirm in studies of additional subjects who had had the same operation.

Some of the new insights that evolved from these studies have occasioned an enormous burgeoning of interest in the left-brain, right-brain phenomenon—among psychologists as well as biologists. In the process, new concepts of consciousness and the workings of the human brain have emerged. Because of increasing public demands for relevance in government-funded science, I am often asked to spell out some of the more practical implications of our neuroscientific investigations in terms of medical perspective and changing views of man and the human mind.

But before I talk about left-brain, right-brain, I must go back a step or two. When we first launched our investigation into the functional role of brain connections, one of the first things we learned was how much we had to *un*learn. At that time, neuroscience was thoroughly sold on the notion that brain function was infinitely malleable. Among other things, the functional interchangeability of nerves in neurosurgery was taken for granted. Having its "wires" crossed by the neurosurgeon supposedly created no problem at all for the brain back in the thirties.

In those days, if any damage was done to a nerve that normally transmits the necessary messages to, say, the muscles of the face, that nerve would be replaced surgically by a nearby healthy and more expendable nerve, such as the one used in lifting the shoulder. The initial effect would be that the face muscles would move whenever the patient tried to lift his shoulder. However, the doctrine of the day prescribed that if the patient went home and practiced in front of a mirror, those malleable brain centers would shortly undergo reeducation to restore normal facial expression, now mediated through the brain centers and nerves designed for shoulder movement.

At the same time, efforts were being made to restore function to legs paralyzed by spinal-cord lesions. The technique involved using one of the main nerves of the *arm* without disconnecting that nerve from the brain centers. The arm nerve was dissected out, full-length, then tunneled under the skin, and connected to the leg nerves so that it would take over the function of the paralyzed limb. Only an early report of this procedure—*not* the final, disappointing outcome—appeared in the literature, for perhaps understandable reasons. Nevertheless, exactly the same operation was later (in the thirties) reported to be a functional success in experimental tests with rats. The motor, the sensory, and even the reflex functions of a paralyzed hind limb were said to have been restored through the transplanted nerves (working via the brain centers) of the forelimb. Thus, even scientists, trying to follow the most objective standards, now and then deceive themselves in the direction of their preconceptions.

In those days the nervous system was generally supposed to be possessed of a wholesale behavioral plasticity or, as one authority put it, "a colossal adaptation capacity almost without limit." The followers of Pavlov in Russia and John Watson in this country were speculating that it should be feasible to shape human nature into virtually any desirable mold and thus to create a more ideal society, by means of appropriate early training and conditioning.

This kind of thinking was reinforced by other views current in the thirties. In particular, the prevalent doctrine concerning nerve growth told us that during embryonic, fetal, and early childhood development, fiber outgrowth and the formation of nerve connections in the

127

brain were essentially diffuse and nonselective. That is, a nerve would connect as readily in one place as it would in another, as in any good standard household wiring system. There seemed to be no way by which the nerve circuits that governed behavior could be grown into the brain directly—that is, *pre*functionally, through inheritance, without being shaped by experience. It was supposed that the adjustment in brain connections depended *entirely* on function and that it began during the earliest movements of the fetus *in utero,* continuing from then on through trial and error, conditioning, learning, experience, through any means but heredity. Our experimental findings in the forties, however, effected a 180-degree about-face in our understanding of these matters. As we now know, nerves are *not* functionally interchangeable. The brain is not all that malleable, and the growth of nerve paths and nerve connections in the brain is anything but diffuse and nonselective. Neural circuits for behavior are definitely grown in, prefunctionally, *under genetic control*—and with great precision in an enormously complex, preprogrammed, biochemically controlled system.

This brief historical review is not just an excuse to recall old times. The point is that while all this has now become a matter of history for those of us in the biomedical sciences, the early views that became so deeply entrenched all through the twenties, thirties, and well into the forties have still not been completely shaken off in other areas. The lingering aftereffect of these doctrines may still be found exerting an unwarranted influence on related disciplines, such as psychiatry, anthropology, and sociology, as well as on society at large. The result is that the majority of us still have a tendency to underrate the genetic and other innate factors in behavior.

What dictates which hemisphere is dominant, whether the individual will be left-handed or right-handed? A recent theory put forth by Jerry Levy of the University of Pennsylvania and Thomas Nagylaki of the University of Wisconsin (both formerly at Cal Tech) proposes that there are two genes governing cerebral dominance and handedness. Each of these two genes has two versions, or "alleles"; thus, there are four in all. One gene determines which hemisphere of the developing brain will be language-dominant, and a second gene determines whether the preferred hand will be on the same side as, or opposite to, the language hemisphere. Without going into the details, if we count up the possible dominant and recessive characteristics contained in these few genes, we come up with nine different combinations of inherited genotypes, each with distinct properties of cerebral dominance and handedness. Some of the left-handers, for instance, will be more resistant than others to reversal by training, because of their genetic pattern.

Now, both the left and right hemispheres of the brain have been found to have their own specialized forms of intellect. The left is highly verbal and mathematical, performing with analytic, symbolic, computerlike, sequential logic. The right, by contrast, is spatial and mute, performing with a synthetic spatio-perceptual and mechanical kind of information processing that cannot yet be simulated by computers. When one is dealing with neurosurgical patients whose left and right hemispheres have been surgically disconnected, it is most impressive and compelling to watch a subject solve a given problem like two different people, in two consistently different ways, using two quite different strategies—depending on whether the subject is using his left or his right hemisphere.

In other words, the nine combinations of genotypes, representing different balancing and loadings of left and right mental factors, provide just in themselves quite a spectrum for inherent individuality in the structure of human intellect. Left-handers as a group have been shown to be different statistically from right-handers in their mental makeup—that is, in IQs and in other test profiles. Similarly, the profiles of males are different from those of females. And females masculinized *in utero* or those lacking one X chromosome are shown to be different from normal females.

Many kinds of tests have shown that the right hemisphere is particularly talented and superior to the left in visual-spatial abilities. This speciality of the so-called minor hemisphere, according to a recent report in the *American Journal of Human Genetics* by Darrell Bock of the University of Chicago and Donald Kolakowski of the University of Connecticut, is tied to a recessive sex-linked gene; that is, a gene linked to the X chromosome, of which the mother has two and the father has only one. In any case, the specialty is shown to exhibit a cross-correlation pattern of inheritance from parents to off-spring in such a clear-cut manner that this aspect of cerebral dominance is seen to be purely genetic, and other theories dealing with environment, experience, or child development as being responsible for it are ruled out.

Because of the distinctly human differences in left-brain, right-brain, and the spectrum of variations that genetic inheritance makes possible in brain physiology—and *therefore* in temperament and talents—each individual brain is truly unique. The degree and kind of inherent individuality each of us carries around in his brain—in its surface features, its internal fiber organization, microstructure, and chemistry—would probably make those differences seen in facial features or in fingerprint patterns look relatively simple and crude by comparison.

A second message that emerges from the findings on hemispheric specialization is that our educational system and modern society generally (with its very heavy emphasis on communication and on early training in the three *R*s) discriminate against one whole half of the

130

brain. I refer, of course, to the nonverbal, nonmathematical, minor hemisphere, which, we find, has its own perceptual, mechanical, and spatial mode of apprehension and reasoning. In our present school system, the attention given to the minor hemisphere of the brain is minimal compared with the training lavished on the left, or major, hemisphere.

A third and final message for social change that we get from the world of the laboratory is a complex one that precludes a simple summary. One of the more important things to come out of our brain research in recent years —from my standpoint, at least—is a greatly changed idea of the conscious mind and its relation to brain mechanism. The new interpretation, or reformulation, involves a direct break with long-established materialistic and behavioristic thinking, which has dominated neuroscience for many decades. Instead of dispensing with consciousness as just an "inner aspect" of the brain process, or as some passive "epiphenomenon" or other impotent by-product, as has been the custom, our present interpretation would make the conscious mind an integral part of the brain process itself and an essential constituent of the action. As a dynamic emergent property of cerebral excitation, subjective experience acquires causal potency and becomes a causal determinant in brain function. Although inseparably tied to the material brain process, it is something distinct and special in its own right, "different from and more than" its component physiochemical elements.

Its directive control influence is seen to reside in the universal power of the whole over its parts, in this case the power of high-order cerebral processes over their constituent neurochemical components. On these new terms, consciousness is put to work, given a use and a reason for being and for having been evolved in a material world. Not only does the brain's physiology determine the mental effects, as has been generally agreed,

131

but now, in addition, the emergent mental operations are conceived in turn to control the component neurophysiology through their higher organizational properties. The scheme provides a conceptual explanatory model for the interaction of mind with matter in terms that do not violate the principles of scientific explanation or those of modern neuroscience.

After more than fifty years of strict behaviorist avoidance of such terms as "mental imagery" and visual, verbal, auditory "images," these terms have, in the past five years, come into wide usage as explanatory constructs in the literature on cognition, perception, and other higher functions.

The revised interpretation brings the conscious mind into the causal sequence in human decision making—and therefore into behavior generally—and thus back into the realm of experimental science, from which it has long been excluded. This swing in psychology and neuroscience away from hard-core materialism and reductionism toward a new, more acceptable brand of mentalism tends now to restore to the scientific image of human nature some of the dignity, freedom, and other humanistic attributes of which it had been deprived by the behavioristic approach.

Old metaphysical dualisms and the seemingly irreconcilable paradoxes that formerly prevailed between the realities of inner experience on the one hand and those of experimental brain science on the other have become reconciled today in a single continuum from the brain's subnuclear particles on up—through atoms and molecules to cells and nerve-circuit systems without consciousness, to cerebral processes with consciousness.

When subjective values are conceived to have objective consequences in the brain, they no longer need to be set off outside the domain of science. The old proposition that science deals with facts, not with values, and its corollary, that value judgments lie outside the realm of science, no longer apply in the new framework. Instead of separating science from values, the present interpretation (when all the various ramifications and logical implications are followed through) leads to a stand in which science becomes the best source, method, and authority for determining ultimate value and those ultimate ethical axioms and guideline beliefs to live and govern by. By the word *science* I refer broadly to the knowledge, understanding, insight, and perspectives that come from science. But, more particularly, I am thinking of the principles for establishing validity and reliability and credibility of the scientific way as an approach to truth, insofar as the human brain can comprehend truth.

AFTERWORD:

Eyes Left! Eyes Right!

James H. Austin

A simple but striking instance of the left-brain, right-brain dichotomy is the way it can affect one's eye movements. The characteristic direction of these movements often yields interesting information about a person's attitudes and ways of thinking.

To test this proposition, in the laboratory, the subject's eyes are observed as he is asked questions that might be handled by either brain hemisphere. One question might be: "If you were President, how would you deal with the Middle East situation?" Or, "What is the meaning of the proverb 'Better a bad peace than a good

---

Dr. James H. Austin is a neuroscientist at the University of Colorado Medical Center.

133

war'?" One observes that the subject's eyes glance (and frequently his head also turns) in one direction as he begins to reflect about the answer. Some look quickly to the left; others look first to the right. The direction of gaze of most persons is reasonably consistent (78 to 80 percent of the time in the same direction). The direction of this initial flickering shift, at the moment of pondering, permits researchers to classify people as "right-movers" or "left-movers."

What kinds of people glance to the left? Those who are more prone to focus on their internal subjective experiences. "Left-movers" are more readily hypnotizable, more likely to have been classical-humanistic majors in college, and are somewhat more likely to report clear visual imagery. It is significant to our understanding of creativity to note that the more readily hypnotizable person is one whose subjective experiences are rich, who accepts impulses from within, and who is capable of deep imaginative involvements.

Who are the right-movers? They tend to major in science or in "hard," quantitative subjects in college, and they are better at mathematical problems than in verbal ability. They are also quicker to identify concepts when the problem is based on words, as in this problem: "What adjective applies to the nouns—sky, ocean, eyes, jeans?"

What does the direction of a glance tell us about the way the brain functions? It implies a physiological bias—a preexisting "set." One hemisphere seems poised to act a fraction of a second before the other. In a sense, the connections of this half of the brain will take the lead in the person's psychophysiological functioning. When you consciously glance at an apple off to your left, you have an external object to look at, and it is activity within your right frontal lobe that starts your eyes moving to the left. But when there is no external target to look at deliberately, the glance is unconscious, spontaneous, determined by internal factors. It is plausible to think, then, that when left-movers start their movement of internal reflection, they are revealing the greater facility in function within their right cerebral hemisphere. This bias in favor of the right hemisphere more readily activates the eye-movement connections of their right frontal lobe and expresses itself in a quick, unconscious glance to the left.

How significant a glance may be as a clue to basic differences among persons in their temperaments, lifestyles, and the way they create can, for the moment, be better imagined than defined, for the basic descriptive work is still going on, and much still needs to be done before we truly understand what is going on, and how. Again, we see that an observation raises far more questions than it answers. But in the interim, the issues raised illustrate the spectrum of decisions—subjective/objective, humanistic/scientific—that our two hemispheres make every day throughout many levels of creative thought.

A vast chorus of internal dialogue, verbal and nonverbal, embellishes our loosest associations as we dream, or focuses our concentrated attention when we are awake. Communication between the two hemispheres of the brain is essential if our creative efforts are to be well integrated in many dimensions: verbal and visual-spatial; internal and external; past, present, and future. Indeed, when the halves of the brain exchange their disparate experiences, pool their viewpoints and approaches, the resulting synthesis brings to problem solving a whole symphony of talents. The corpus callosum serves as the major thoroughfare rapidly transferring this information. Through it the left hemisphere speaks, quite literally, to the right, and the right hemisphere answers, *sotto voce,* with its own repertoire of musical refrains or visual metaphors.

Because the frontal, parietal, temporal, occipital, and

limbic lobes of the brain are each paired, we begin to see the whole creative quest as the fusion of a major orchestral performance, with drum beats and clashing cymbals from all the more primitive deeper structures of the brain stem contributing their basic rhythm and passion to the score.

Observing the Brain
Through a Cat's Eyes

by Roger Lewin

What does a baby see when it gazes out on the world around itself? Does it see pretty much what its parents see? Or does each baby see a "mud-luscious, puddle-wonderful" world quite different from the one its parents—and for that matter, all other babies—are looking at?

Scientists and philosophers have argued this question of vision since Aristotle's day. But now researchers experimenting on cats have made revolutionary discoveries about the way we see—discoveries that apply not only to cats but also to the people who feed them.

The main revelation is that the ability to "see straight" does not develop in children automatically, that is, quite apart from any outside influences. Instead, the researchers have found, our visual machinery is strongly shaped by our early experiences—experiences that drastically affect the way we see the world in later life and that may even determine how gifted we will be musically and linguistically. It may be that areas of great potential in child

Dr. Roger Lewin is life-science editor of the British magazine *New Scientist.*

development are being wasted simply because we don't teach the right things at the right time, the time when children's brains are most receptive.

The pioneers of the vision research on cats are two Harvard biologists, David Hubel and Torsten Wiesel. When they began their study, in the early sixties, they expected to find that a cat's early environment has some small shaping influence on the way its vision develops. But like all the other biologists now interested in the work, Hubel and Wiesel have been absolutely amazed by the remarkable flexibility and plasticity displayed by the cat's visual system as it slowly develops. It now appears possible to persuade nerve cells in the cat's brain to do jobs for which they were never designed. Even if the rest of the brain is capable of only a fraction of the plasticity evident in the workings of the visual cortex, there is still a great deal of scope for external influences affecting the way the brain develops.

In the beginning Hubel and Wiesel looked at the activity of nerve cells in the so-called primary area of the visual cortex. These cells turned out to be "feature detectors"—that is, they respond to specific shapes seen by the eye. Generally, there are two types of feature detectors: the ones that are found in many animal species and others that are specific to a particular species. These latter usually enable the animal to flourish in its behavioral environment. For instance, the frog has visual cells that are almost lightheartedly called "bug detectors"; these react when an object the size of a fly enters the animal's field of vision. One can argue that these specific feature detectors are programmed genetically, but it is also tempting to think that they may be at least partly shaped by early environmental influence.

The feature detectors, which Hubel and Wiesel located by means of minute electrodes pushed into the adult cat's brain, turned out to be orientation-selective; that is, they respond to—or, in scientific terms, are "specific to"—any line or edge moving across the animal's visual field along a particular orientation or angle. Any one cell is specific to a particular orientation, but all angles through the entire range of 360 degrees are "covered" by the population of nerve cells in this area of the brain. The Harvard team also discovered that most of the cells here are binocular, or wired up to both eyes.

In contrast to the adult cat, the visually naïve kitten has practically no mature feature detectors. The cells are certainly present in the brain, but they have not yet been recruited to their job. The binocular connections in the kitten are just like the adult's. In one of Hubel and Wiesel's early experiments to try to discover the forces (genetic or environmental) that convert an infant eye to an adult one, they kept a growing kitten in total darkness and then examined its brain. They discovered that the binocular wiring had remained intact, but that the feature detectors had suffered terribly, remaining very immature. Here was a strong indication of environmental input determining brain development.

Next, Hubel and Wiesel tried covering just one of an animal's eyes to see what that does to the brain. This time the feature detectors worked fine, but the binocular connections were thrown awry; they had all gone to the one seeing eye. Hubel and Wiesel found that the visual brain was plastic only during a "sensitive period" of the animal's life: from three weeks to three months. Again, this fits in with the notion that early experience is important in brain development.

The obvious implications of this work for an understanding of human development soon drew other research teams in to probe the problems, and the results have been astounding. For instance, Colin Blakemore and his colleagues in Cambridge, England, have found that in a visually inexperienced kitten they can induce the switch from inbuilt binocularity to monocularity after just *six* hours' vision through one eye. The change isn't

139

made immediately; a period of consolidation is required following the programming exposure. Blakemore likens this response to learning and memory: in learning, an experience is slotted into a temporary store (short-term memory), and then a more permanent record is made (long-term memory).

The binocular/monocular switch is even more re-markable because it can be repeated again and again. If first one eye is covered, and then the other, and so on, the brain connections with the eyes will switch each time to the seeing eye, but once again this elaborate neural dance is possible only during the sensitive period.

The most remarkable results come from the plasticity of the feature detectors. Following up the early Harvard experiments, Colin Blakemore and Graham Cooper at Cambridge and Nico Spinelli and Helmut Hirsch at Stanford hit on the same idea: to put visually naïve kittens into artificial environments to see if the feature detectors can be manipulated. It turns out that they can.

For instance, the Cambridge kittens were reared in visual environments consisting only of vertical stripes *or* horizontal stripes, not both. When the animals emerged from their striped worlds into the real visual world, they behaved in a most extraordinary way. "Horizontal" cats were perfectly capable of jumping onto a chair to settle down for a sleep; but when walking on the floor, they kept bumping into the chair legs, just as if the legs were invisible. In contrast, "vertical" animals had no difficulty in negotiating the chair-leg hazards, but they never tried to jump onto a chair; it was as if the seat were not there.

When the Blakemore team looked inside the kittens' heads, the animals' curious behavior was explained at once. The vertical cats had no horizontal-feature detectors; so they literally could not see anything that was composed of horizontal lines, like the seat of a chair. And the horizontal animals had only horizontal detectors, which made it impossible for them to see the vertical chair legs. These animals really were blind to things in their environment that were perfectly visible to you and me and to any self-respecting cat, all because of their unusual early experience.

This curious saga gets more curious still. Very recently Blakemore and his team, and California researchers Jack Pettigrew and Horace Barlow, managed to pervert all of the orientation detectors in cats: the researchers made the detectors respond to spots, not lines—something that the cells were never "designed" to do. The trick was simply to bring up the animals in a spotty environment rather than a stripy one. Electrodes probed into the animals' brains revealed that it was spots displayed in the visual field that excited the cells in the visual cortex, not lines as in normal animals. Because the animals have to create a picture of their external world by synthesizing the responses of these nerve cells, it is anyone's guess what the unfortunate felines actually "saw" when they emerged—probably a fuzzy, hazy picture, somewhat like fog.

Blakemore and Don Mitchell, a colleague from Dalhousie University, Canada, decided to measure the speed at which the character of the feature detectors is specified. The researchers were more than astounded at the result, for they discovered that, with as little as one hour's visual experience, the way an animal's feature detectors function can be pretty well changed. The analogy with learning again enters one's mind.

Most people now agree that the cat's "visual-sensitive" period falls within the three-week-to-three-month span that Hubel and Wiesel noticed, with the most sensitive time occurring at about five weeks. This makes good developmental sense, because it is at this time that the animal's eyes have just about swung around to their correct positions in the sockets and the fluid within the eyes

141

has become clear. But what about humans? Is there the same plasticity? If so, is there a sensitive period? If so, when is it?

Inevitably, the evidence for humans has to be rather more indirect than it has been for cats, but the indications are that there is not much difference between us and our feline cousins. For instance, infants with uncorrected squint or severe astigmatism finish up with permanent defects; spectacles cannot help them because it is the brain that appears to be at fault, not the eyes. In contrast, astigmatism that develops in adulthood can be corrected optically. This indicates that, like the brain of the cat, the immature human brain *is* plastic, while the adult brain is not. Blakemore says that the human visual-sensitive period probably spans the years from two to four. Visual defects really should be corrected before then.

Possibly the most intriguing discovery in this whole tale has come just recently from Canadian researchers Robert Annis and Barrie Frost. They examined the visual abilities of city-dwellers and compared them with those of Cree Indians living in tepees on the east coast of James Bay. In the past, researchers had found that "normal" people have better visual acuity (can see most sharply) in the horizontal and vertical axes. But what Annis and Frost found throws into question this concept of normality. They discovered that the Cree Indians have no particular axis of high visual acuity and are not especially attuned to horizontal and vertical lines. These people had, of course, been brought up in the country and away from the city, which is dominated by rectangular shapes. It may well be that the normal horizontal and vertical visual-acuity preferences are imposed on us simply because we live in a rectangular world. If houses were spherical instead of boxlike, things might be different. The crucial point is that human vision does appear to display the same kind of plasticity found in the experimental cats. And what is true of vision probably applies to our other senses as well.

Pediatricians have long recognized that infants should not be closeted in drab, visually unstimulating nurseries; the work with cats now gives that intuitive realization some scientific backing. But can we go further than this? Will a child become a musical genius if he is bombarded with Beethoven, Bach, and Berlioz from the day he is born? Will talking to a child in a spectrum of languages enhance his linguistic talent? And will one be the parent of a great mathematician if one teaches his infant the elements of logic at a tender age? The answer to all of these is, probably, "up to a point."

Almost certainly, the learning capacity of the human brain has not been exploited to the full by current educational approaches. The essential point is the possible existence of sensitive periods, not just for visual development but for music, language, logic, and artistic talents. For instance, everyone acquires the elements of his language between the ages of two and four. So why wait another six years before teaching a child a second and third language? The brain is clearly attuned to language acquisition in the early years, and there is a lot of evidence about the ease with which youngsters pick up foreign languages to which they are exposed. It would probably be a mistake to try to teach children two languages at once when they are only two years old, because there would be retroactive interference between the languages. But a child of four could start on a new language.

Musical talent very often runs in families. It may be "in the genes," of course, but there is undoubtedly a large environmental element, too. Children exposed to a lot of music when young are almost always more musically talented than average; how much this development is due to encouragement and opportunity is difficult to tell. But evidence that the musical brain becomes keyed in to its early experiences comes from the observation that people who develop perfect pitch while exposed to a slightly out-of-tune instrument always match their pitch to the instrument's. Although playing Beethoven to one's infant will probably not cause an environmentally generated reincarnation of the grand master, it may well produce a more-than-usually musically talented child.

Probably the most important skill that children learn is *how* to learn. The mark of intelligence is the facility for solving problems. Too often we give children answers to remember rather than problems to solve. This is a mistake. Unless children develop the art of problem solving —whether by analytical logic or by nonsequential intuition—their brains will remain underexploited. Everyone knows that infants go through a period of being intensely curious. This curiosity is probably a behavioral expression of the brain's most sensitive period for acquiring knowledge and learning techniques.

Researchers will now turn their minds to discovering more about specific sensitive periods in the development of the brain, whether for language acquisition, enhancing musical talent, or simply learning how to learn. Unless these periods are exploited to the full at the right time, their potential may be lost forever.

AFTERWORD:

How Real Is

Our Reality?

by Albert Rosenfeld

I am haunted by the experiments described in Roger Lewin's article. Two groups of kittens are trained in separate, carefully controlled environments. One group can perceive only horizontal lines while the other sees only vertical ones. When both groups move out into the real world, we are treated to the disquieting spectacle of two sets of intelligent animals, both of the same species (they could even be siblings), both perfectly normal (within the definition of their upbringing); each sharing the same reality, yet experiencing that reality in a radically different manner—each, in fact, quite blind to important segments of the other's universe.

One can easily imagine a society where the horizontal-oriented cats were in the overwhelming majority and in unequivocal political ascendancy. Their view of the world would of course represent the norm. Those few cats who perceived vertically would be "hallucinating." They might be adjudged insane and put away in the crazy-cage. Verticality might even be considered subversive or heretical.

"What is reality?" is a question as old as philosophy. Even ancient sages understood, long before scientific insight made it explicitly clear, that our reality is closely related to our biology (especially to our neurobiology), to the ways in which we perceive.

Suppose ten of us are in a room, and I take a dose of LSD. In a short time I will be seeing and sensing all kinds of bizarre and distorted visions—all very real to me. But inasmuch as your view of the world remains unchanged, I am hallucinating. The electrochemistry of my brain cells and fluids has been scrambled in such a way as to distort all my "normal" perceptions. But suppose it were possible to scramble the brains of all ten of us simultaneously in precisely the same detailed manner, so that we were all hallucinating together. Might our hallucinations then be identified as real—especially if we didn't suspect that our brains had been meddled with?

Through the centuries, philosophers have grappled with the problem of a reality we can count on—the "something-I-know-not-what" that John Locke was sure must underlie our perceptions. Or could reality be, as Bishop Berkeley argued, merely an idea in the mind of

God? If a hypnotist can put ten people into a trance simultaneously and suggest to them an event—thus making it real for them, even though we "know" it "didn't really happen"—why couldn't an omnipotent mind, if one existed, similarly impose its own reality on the minds of a whole population or of a whole species?

We do of course realize, even if only by analogy, that perception has limits. We know that the mole and the dragonfly see a different world from the one we see. (They may not see at all, in the strict human sense.) We know, too, that reality exists beyond the reach of our senses—sound waves past the threshold of our audibility, electromagnetic radiations stretching far on both sides of the narrow spectral slit visible to our eyes.

We also recognize that we can't always accept the evidence of our senses. To us, the Earth appears flat; the stars are pinpoints of light fixed on the dark roof of night; a rock is a dense, motionless solid rather than a mostly empty space sparsely populated by dancing atoms, seemingly "at rest" on a round, unresting Earth, itself a speck of cosmic dust lost in the unimaginable vastnesses of galaxies in nonstop flight.

"What is reality?" is, then, a question difficult to answer in any absolute way. On a commonsense, everyday level, we don't usually need to trouble ourselves with such abstruse considerations. As a practical matter, we settle for what our senses report—as long as the senses of others report the same things. Ordinary reality, then, is consensual reality—reality by consensus.

Let's go back to the ten of us in a room and skip the LSD. If I point to a table, a book, a chandelier, and you all see these objects, their reality will not be questioned. If I say I saw a bird fly through the room, and if no one else saw it, you will think that I am either lying or hallucinating. If a bird really does fly through the room, and if I succeed, through hypnosis, in erasing the event from your minds—though your testimony outweighs mine by nine to one—I am the one who knows what really happened. On the other hand, if I could hypnotize you into accepting a totally imaginary bird flight, you would all swear to the reality you had "seen."

Sheer sophistry? Maybe so. After all, who would have any *reason* to be playing the cosmic jokester, to be tricking us this way all the time? Besides, there must be very few people in the world who have such hypnotic powers (I surely have not). Nevertheless, these are good, instructive "thought games" to play as a reminder of how plastic and suggestible are our minds and our perceptions.

The most pertinent questions that the horizontal and vertical cats give rise to are: How much of our reality is imprinted on us by our culture? How much is denied us? We are taught what we are taught when we are at our most pliant, long before we have anything to say about it. In the process, what worlds are lost to us? Many creative people in the contemporary human-potential movements are convinced that (just as don Juan is supposed to have demonstrated to Carlos Castaneda) other realities exist beyond our usual perceptions—realities we could have access to if only we could learn to open ourselves up to them.

Like the horizontally deprived cats, do we blunder around the world, never seeing beautiful places where we might stretch out and ease our souls? Like the missing verticals, do we keep knocking ourselves silly against obstacles we can't see are there?

The Promise and Peril
of Psychosurgery

by Richard Restak

Psychosurgery is a term used rather broadly these days to describe surgical, electrical, and other alterations of the brain to change human behavior. An important distinguishing feature of any psychosurgical procedure is irreversibility. Once the brain tissue is altered, it can never be the same again. Since the brain is the essence of what we refer to as personality, it follows that psychosurgery irrevocably alters personality. Even at its best, therefore, psychosurgery is the most hazardous form of psychiatric treatment yet devised and currently the most controversial.

Experts in medicine, behavior, ethics, and law have clashed over the most fundamental question in the field: Who should designate candidates for psychosurgery and for what symptoms? Should a brain operation to reduce aggression, say, be recommended by a neurologist? A psychiatrist? A social worker? This confusion is inherent in our primitive understanding of the way the brain functions. Since we do not know how it performs "normally," we are even more at a loss to predict how it will perform after surgery. Some examples:

- In San Francisco, a fifty-five-year-old minister suffering from an incurably painful cancer undergoes

148

"psychosurgery." In three months he returns free of pain to the pulpit, after an absence of four years.
• In Jackson, Mississippi, a psychosurgeon operates on a fourteen-year-old boy with explosively violent behavior. After the surgery the boy is withdrawn and cannot remember his address. After further operations he is described as "deteriorated intellectually."

Recently the National Institute of Mental Health sponsored a conference on psychosurgery. Appearing by invitation was Dr. O. J. Andy, director of neurosurgery at the University of Mississippi School of Medicine in Jackson. Dr. Andy, perhaps this country's leading proponent of psychosurgery as a solution to the problem of chronic psychiatric disease, explained his position to the conferees:

All abnormal behavior results from structurally abnormal brain tissue. Now, psychiatric techniques are in most instances futile in dealing with these abnormalities. In fact, adequate therapy can be obtained only by techniques, such as surgery, which deal directly with the structurally abnormal brain tissue. [When pressed on this point, Dr. Andy is willing to admit that no one has demonstrated abnormalities in the structure of brain tissue in psychiatric disease.] It is unfortunate that our institutions are constantly filled with patients having behavioral disorders which do not respond to psychiatric and medical therapy and which would respond to surgery but are denied appropriate treatment for a variety of rational and irrational reasons. My own clinical interest has been in the realm of controlling aggressive, uncontrollable, violent, and hyperactive behavior which does not respond to medical or psychiatric therapy. I have developed a clinical description of such behavior: the Hyperresponsive Syndrome. This is erratic, aggressive, hyperactive, and emotional instability which in its full-blown expression terminates in attack. These are the patients who need surgical treatment. In addition, there are others: patients who are a detriment to themselves and to society; custodial patients who require constant attention, supervision, and an inordinate amount of institutional care. It should be used in children and adolescents in order to allow their developing brain to mature with as normal a reaction to its environment as possible.

Dr. Andy went on to explain that many of his subjects have been children aged seven and over; at least one was a child of five. The goal in each case is "to reduce the hyperactivity to levels manageable by parents."

The exact number of operations performed by Dr. Andy lies between forty and fifty, but he is not sure exactly how many. Moreover, several children have had more than one operation; in at least one case, five different operations were required in order to bring about "behavioral control."

At one point in Dr. Andy's address he was interrupted by a question regarding the medical ethics of his psychosurgical procedures. He replied:

The ethics involved in the treatment of behavioral disorders is no different from the ethics involved in the treatment of all medical disorders. The medical problems involving behavior have a more direct impact on society than other medical problems such as coronary or kidney disease. Still, if treatment is desired, it is neither the moral nor the legal responsibility of society [to determine] what type of treatment should be administered. The ethics for the diagnosis and treatment of behavioral illness should remain in the hands of the treating physician.

The concept of modifying behavior by surgically cutting parts of the brain is not new. First references to such a procedure can be traced to the Roman observation that insanity might be relieved by a sword wound in the head. But all modern psychosurgical methods date from physiologist James Fulton's observation that cutting a specialized group of nerve fibers from the frontal lobes of the brains of two chimpanzees, Becky and Lucy, led to a taming of the animals. The chimps could remember old tricks, even learn new ones, but accepted test situations and frustrations with a "philosophical calm."

In 1936 Egas Moniz, a Portuguese neurologist, applied a similar technique to uncontrollable psychotics. Thirteen years later Moniz won a Nobel Prize and was commended for "the development of prefrontal leucotomy in the treatment of certain psychoses." The number of lobotomies, as this procedure came to be called, performed by Moniz is unknown. Any exact computation is complicated by Moniz's early retirement from neurologic practice several years before a violent death at the hands of a crazed former patient.

In 1942 Walter Freeman, a neurologist, and James Watts, a neurosurgeon, both at George Washington University Hospital, reported that extreme depression and agitation, even hallucination, could be greatly alleviated by cutting the fibers leading from the frontal lobes of the brain to the neighboring thalamus. The connections between these two structures are normally responsible for a delicate interplay between thought (a frontal-lobe function) and emotion (at least partly a thalamic function). After cutting these connections, the doctors reported that exaggerated emotional responses decreased. Although in some cases hallucinations continued, they were far less terrifying.

The Freeman–Watts treatment spread quickly, and during the 1940s somewhere in the range of 50,000 patients were lobotomized in the United States alone. Freeman, a lobotomy zealot, calculated that he had personally performed over 4,000 operations, using a gold-plated ice pick, which he carried with him in a velvet-lined case. After the local application of a mild painkiller, Freeman would plunge the ice pick through the thin bone of the upper inner angle of the eye socket, severing the frontal nerve connections to the thalamus. No elaborate preparations or precautions preceded this grisly operation, which often took place in the patient's home or in Freeman's office at St. Elizabeth's Hospital in Washington, D.C. Freeman's enthusiasm for "ice-pick surgery" knew no bounds; several former associates, who prefer to remain unnamed, can recall long lines of patients waiting for treatment outside Freeman's office.

Unfortunately, these lobotomies, especially as practiced by Freeman, often resulted in a zombie-like state known as the "frontal-lobe syndrome." Common symptoms included indifference to other people, convulsive seizures, and intellectual impairment. Patients often became self-centered and utterly dependent on others for the simplest routines of day-to-day living.

During the succeeding thirty years, psychosurgeons developed a less crude method of eliminating undesired emotional responses. This involved tampering with the limbic system, or emotional brain—the target of present-day psychosurgery. The limbic system, though still not totally defined, includes such areas as the hippocampus, the amygdala, the cingulum, and the hypothalamus. In lower animals these structures form the basis for emotional reactions. Tampering with the amygdala, for instance, produces in an animal drowsiness, indifference to surroundings, loss of appetite, and a peculiar symptom known as psychic blindness. The animal may stare for hours at food, not realizing it is meant to be eaten. Studies of the human limbic system have established the existence of emotional centers similar in structure, and presumably in function, to those of lower animals. Proponents argue that operations on these limbic areas produce less "blunting" of the personality than is caused by lobotomies.

With the discovery of tranquilizers in the early fifties, interest in surgery on both the frontal lobes and the limbic system declined sharply. A drug called Thorazine was widely used as a kind of chemical lobotomy. It soon became apparent, however, that the use of this "miracle drug" carried its own penalties, particularly drug allergies, serious blood abnormalities, paradoxical reactions resulting in further excitement rather than calm, and a bizarre disorder of muscle tone and movement known as tardive dyskinesia. These failures resulted in a resurgence of interest in psychosurgery.

In the last twenty years at least eight different surgical procedures have been developed in which surgical incisions are made in one or more portions of the limbic system. The two most common operations performed today are cingulotomies and amygdalotomies, which involve deep cuts into these two key areas of the emotional brain. According to limbic-system theory, disturbed emotional patterns (violence, deep depressions, suicidal tendencies, etc.) are partly the result of a form of "short-circuitry" between the limbic system and the rest of the brain. Cutting of the amygdala or the cingulum is intended to interrupt these faulty "connections" in the hope that new "connections" will develop or that the interruption will abolish the disturbed behavior patterns. In actuality, the correlation between behavior patterns and limbic structures is at best disputable.

Surgical advances in the last fifteen years have led to increasingly precise "targets" within the limbic system. The most innovative development involves stereotactic surgery, a revolutionary treatment for Parkinson's disease in the days before the discovery of the drug L-Dopa. Stereotaxis involves the use of a tiny probe guided externally through a small opening made in the skull. By three-dimensional visualization, tiny, accurate cuts can be made in any part of the brain. This procedure markedly reduces the incidence of complications. In many instances ultrasonic beams and radioactive substances have also been used to destroy brain tissue thought to be responsible for emotionally disturbed behavior.

A major advance in the last five years has been the use of small electrodes to stimulate parts of the limbic system. Because the patient is awake, the effects produced by electric stimulation can be described by the patient. If a certain area is found to produce the symptoms for which treatment is sought (rage, depression, etc.), that area can be destroyed. This method has been used for years with good results in the treatment of epilepsy. Its value in treating behavioral disorders, however, has never been established.

Publications regarding psychosurgical operations number many thousands by now. They are, for the most part, contradictory, confusing, and marred by the absence of scientific objectivity. Yet, despite the confusion, contradictions, and, occasionally, downright deception, certain facts have emerged. For one thing, tampering with the frontal fibers is almost certain to produce indifference and apathy. Secondly, certain patients have reacted poorly to psychosurgery regardless of the type of operation. Schizophrenics have done worst of all and have been eliminated from the patient pool of even the most enthusiastic of psychosurgeons. So-called psychopaths or sociopaths have not done much better. In fact, the number of patients who stand to gain from psychosurgical procedures turns out to be remarkably small. It includes severe obsessive-compulsives, such as perpetual hand washers, who may excoriate their hands and arms by two or three hundred washings a day, and a limited number of severe and unremitting depressives who, failing to respond to antidepressant medications or even to electroconvulsive therapy, gravitate toward inevitable suicide. In addition, psychosurgery may help the terminal cancer patient whose mind is never entirely freed from a totally pain-ridden, drug-addicted existence.

Beyond these few cases, however, lies considerable evidence that the procedure is more often dangerous and even irresponsibly applied. At least one West Coast neurosurgeon, for example, has taken to performing psychosurgery on children as an office procedure. As a result of such abuses, psychosurgery is under challenge as a violation of medical ethics and the individual patient's civil rights. Despite this, there exists no binding standards by which psychosurgery can be regulated.

The most pointed legal objection to psychosurgery revolves on loopholes in the present structure of "informed consent": the extent to which the patient has been informed regarding all possible consequences of psychosurgery. Dr. Harold Edgar, associate professor of law at Columbia University Law Center and author of a forthcoming book on psychosurgery, writes:

> As things stand now, the surgeon is covered as long as he explains to the patient and relatives the uncertainties in the methods and gets them to agree to it without guarantee. It is quite possible that some families would be willing to consent to almost anything to get a troublesome relative off their hands. There must be protection against the collusion of such families with overzealous psychosurgeons. The unwilling patient's right must be safeguarded.

The case of obtaining informed consent from prisoners is even more sensitive. Robert C. Neville, of the State University of New York at Purchase, cites the case of "Thomas the Engineer," who was asked to submit to a behavior-control experiment:

155

When under the influence of calming electrical stimulation, he consented to a psychosurgical procedure to destroy certain brain cells. When the effects of the stimulus wore off, he refused consent. What is informed rational consent in such a setting?

The question came to a court test recently, and the decision clarified the ambiguous legal position of psychosurgery. A Michigan court ruled that state funds could not be used to finance psychosurgery on mental patients despite the patient's willingness—even enthusiasm—to undergo the procedure. The patient, convicted eighteen years ago for the rape and subsequent slaying of a nurse, was judged criminally insane and committed to Ionia State Hospital in Detroit. His eligibility for discharge notwithstanding, he requested psychosurgery to eliminate the possibility of losing control and killing again. No coercion was brought to bear; the operation was not a precondition to release.

Still, the voluntary nature of the consent was questioned by attorney Charles Halpern of the Center for Law and Social Policy at the Society of the Neurosciences in Washington. "There is simply no way," he said, "to ensure that a person in the hospital for eighteen years, with a likelihood of imprisonment for more time, can ever make a voluntary judgment on whether he should have this operation."

During court hearings Dr. Ayub Ommaya, director of the research section of the National Institute of Neurologic Diseases and Stroke, also questioned the scientific premise of the proposed electrode operation. "The role of psychosurgery," Ommaya testified, "has little, if any, applicability for violent behavior."

A similar, federal-level setback for psychosurgery occurred on June 26, 1973. The National Institutes of Health rejected a $1.2-million-grant proposal by Dr. Vernon Mark of Harvard and other doctors who pioneered the use of amygdalotomy to treat violent or irrational behavior. The work of the Boston group, in fact, had provided much of the incentive for the Michigan program. Mark and his colleagues had advocated the idea that much crime and other violence have their roots in medical, rather than social, causes—a concept that had already won them grant money from the Nixon administration.

According to Dr. Edgar, the definition of psychosurgery as an experimental process could resolve some ambiguities. This would require additional safety and quantitative procedures, such as the maintenance of control groups, which are not currently observed. A bill providing guidelines for all human experimentation has been introduced in Congress by Senator Edward Kennedy.

The issue of behavior modification is perhaps the century's most compelling medical-social issue. Current fads for ESP and biofeedback reflect our enthusiasm for controlling mental processes with techniques similar to those for controlling our physical environment. Psychosurgery, the most extreme and dramatic form of such modification, involves particularly anguishing decisions that must be made now. Unfortunately, the issue is becoming so politicized that reasoning based on facts is seriously hampered. On December 27, 1972, for example, an open session on psychosurgery and behavioral control at the American Association for the Advance of Science in Washington was disrupted by demonstrators.

In light of such profound disagreements, certain measures seem justified:

1. It is time for a temporary moratorium on all forms of psychosurgery undertaken primarily to modify behavior.

2. We need a clearinghouse of information on the topic of the effects of brain lesions on behavior. As things

now stand, the facts are scattered in hundreds of journals. The clearinghouse would enable the evaluation of the data already accumulated from twenty years of various psychosurgical procedures.

3. From here it should be possible to determine national standards of practice concerning (a) when and if psychosurgery is indicated, (b) what procedures offer reasonable hope of result, and (c) most important, which patients are eligible for psychosurgery and under what circumstances.

4. There is an urgent need for measures that will protect the individual patient from having psychosurgical procedures imposed upon him against his will or in a setting in which informed consent or the capacity to choose is impaired.

5. Since the results of psychosurgery have not been established, all psychosurgical procedures should be considered "experimental" and subject to strictly imposed controls. Such operations should be carried out only in a clinical institution able to provide total therapeutic care and follow-up. Nonmedical disciplines must have significant influence in the control of psychosurgery.

Some critics have suggested that we immediately outlaw psychosurgery altogether. But even this isn't as simple as it seems. What is to be done for tortured compulsives whose senseless rituals defy treatment by any other form? What of the terminal cancer patient whose personality threatens to shatter under the daily strain of unendurable pain? What of the patient who refers himself for a psychosurgical procedure? What are his rights in a possible setting of controlled and reasonably predictable operations? At this point these questions cannot be answered, for want of the facts. Only by implementing measures similar to those listed above can we make a good case to abandon—or expand—the use of psychosurgery.

AFTERWORD:

The Need Is
to Know More, Not Less

by Albert Rosenfeld

Research is at the very heart of science. Merely to report the results of research, however—fascinating as they may be—is not enough. Whoever reports science is also obliged to interpret and evaluate, to maintain a steady radar scan for its impact on our everyday lives. Research has consequences, immediate as well as long-run. These consequences must always be kept in mind, with a view to ensuring—whenever new knowledge leaves the lab and clinic to be applied to the real world and its inhabitants—that the risks do not outweigh the benefits.

In the case of psychosurgery, do we know enough yet about either the risks or the benefits? Is it ethical, in any event, to use the knife as therapy in cases where the couch has failed? These are some of the questions Richard Restak examines in his article.

The immediate moral controversy focuses on the treatment of mental patients. But there are more profound and long-range implications inherent in the new capabilities of psychosurgery. They, along with drugs and other techniques, seem to make possible nothing less than the complete control of human behavior—individually and en masse.

Take, for example, the form of psychosurgery known as ESB (electrical stimulation of the brain), where tiny electrodes are implanted in various regions of the brain and are connected to a terminal that is either cemented into the skull or implanted under the skin. By pushing buttons on a radio transmitter, the researcher can, by remote control, stimulate any area of the brain.

It is fascinating, and a bit frightening, to sit in the laboratory of a brain researcher and watch an experiment on a monkey wired up for ESB. The experimenter, by pushing the appropriate button, can make the monkey feel hot or cold, regardless of surrounding temperature; can make it feel hungry, thirsty, or sated—whether it has just finished a meal or hasn't eaten for days; can make it fearless—or fearful, upset, and anxious—or serene and contented; can make it fall asleep or wake up; can turn its sexual desires on or off at will.

The experimenter can render an animal violently aggressive, or put it in a state of euphoria, merely by stimulating the brain's "pleasure centers." The human brain seems to experience similar generalized pleasures, which have been described as "combining the mystic raptures of the saints with the fleshly raptures of the sinners."

ESB is neither painful nor unpleasant. In fact, the person being stimulated has no way of knowing, unless he is told, that he is under the influence of ESB. The stimulated thought or act is indistinguishable from the spontaneous occurrence of his normal thoughts or actions. This is one aspect of psychosurgery that makes many people apprehensive about the prospect of brain control in our future.

Some human beings have already had the odd experience of controlling their own brains, to a limited extent, via an ESB technique known as ICSS (intracranial self-stimulation). Dr. Robert Heath, of Tulane University, has implanted electrodes into damaged areas of an epileptic patient's brain and furnished him with his own push-button control gadget to carry around. Whenever the patient feels the bare beginnings of a convulsive attack, he can turn it off by pressing a button.

Such devices might conceivably be used in the future for a variety of purposes: to put yourself to sleep or to wake up; to dull your appetite if you want to lose weight; to warm or cool you; to quiet anxiety or make you braver; to turn sexual feelings on or off. Would it be a good thing for people to be able to exercise these controls so easily?

Fortunately, formally established institutes now exist for the sole purpose of dealing with exactly such ethical questions—not only for psychosurgery but for the whole range of possibilities opened up by the biomedical revolution of the last two decades as well.

Emphasis in Restak's article is on the hazards of applying the results of research too soon or too casually. Obviously this kind of early-warning surveillance is essential to our welfare. But we must also guard against falling into the reverse trap: Whenever the negative aspects of research are emphasized, there is an uncritical tendency in some quarters to equate science itself with evil, to talk of curtailing research efforts as being more troublesome than beneficial.

But there is nothing about science (or scientific research) in itself that is morally reprehensible. Science is, at worst, neutral. The good or evil resides in the uses we make of it.

Knowing too much is *not* our problem today. At this critical juncture in our planet's history, there is hardly an area of major concern—pollution, overpopulation, the energy crisis, the killer diseases, the sources of violent behavior, the mechanics of peacekeeping—about which we don't need to know *more* than we now know.

The best hope of acquiring the knowledge and understanding we will need to solve our urgent and complex contemporary dilemmas is through intelligent research —not decelerated but, rather, moving full speed ahead.

Irving Cooper:
Pacemakers for the Brain
by David Hendin

Beneath the decaying skeleton of New York City's Third Avenue El at 183d Street in the Bronx stands the entrance to St. Barnabas Hospital for Chronic Diseases. Once called St. Barnabas Hospital for Incurables, the institution today is a far from hopeless place for many of its patients.

Over the past twenty years nearly 10,000 patients at the hospital and thousands more around the world have been given relief from crippling diseases through surgical techniques developed by Dr. Irving Spencer Cooper, a St. Barnabas neurosurgeon. At fifty, Dr. Cooper has to his credit more significant innovations in brain surgery than any other man alive. Recently, according to the *Journal of the American Medical Association,* Cooper has added "another bead—perhaps the largest yet—to his string of achievements in functional neurosurgery." This "biggest bead" is an ingenious device that delivers elec-

---

David Hendin, nationally syndicated health columnist, is the author of *Death As a Fact of Life* and *The Life-Givers*.

162

trical impulses to the cerebellum.* In many cases, this "pacemaker" stops the disabling seizures of previously intractable epilepsy, reduces the spasticity of cerebral-palsy victims, and eases the spastic paralysis that often follows a stroke.

During the past fourteen months, Cooper has implanted his cerebellar stimulator, with varying degrees of success, in about fifty patients. None of the patients has had any adverse effects from the procedure, which, unlike most brain operations, does not destroy part of the brain itself. The surgery consists simply of placing over the front and rear of the cerebellum the system's two sets of silicone-coated, Dacron-enmeshed platinum electrodes. Wires are then run under the skin and down the neck to the chest, where two receivers are embedded. Over this spot the surgeon tapes a battery-powered radio transmitter the size of a cigarette pack. When activated, the transmitter sends a small current through the cerebellum, an inhibitory part of the brain that functions somewhat like a rheostat, and regulates certain of its activities.

"We theorize," says Cooper, "that cerebellar stimulation is modulating the central nervous system in these patients. The effect is different in each case; that is, activity (electrical stimulation) is corrected according to the patient's needs."

One of Cooper's former neurology professors at the Mayo Clinic, Reginald Bickford, who is now at the University of California at San Diego, confirms that "this is very important work. Not only is it possible to abort

---

*The brain pacemaker as a theoretical concept, utilizing a beat-frequency oscillator similar in principle to that developed by Dr. Cooper, was put forth independently in a 1959 publication, "Extending Vision With Electronics," by Dr. F. J. G. Van den Bosch, a Belgian biophysicist now at the Downstate Medical Center in Brooklyn, New York.

epileptic seizures, but unexpectedly this seems to change the tendency even to have seizures. The surgery might also lead to research on drugs that accomplish the same thing. And it is important because it will tell us more about the brain."

The $3,000 brain-pacemaker system, which is still being improved, was conceived by Cooper and developed by him and engineer Roger Avery.

The groundwork for Irving Cooper's career was laid in 1952, when, as an assistant professor of surgery at New York University, he performed an established operation on a Parkinson's patient. His intent was to cut the motor pathway in the midbrain, thus swapping the victim's shaking palsy for partial paralysis. During the delicate operation, the young surgeon accidentally tore open the tiny anterior choroidal artery that leads to two motor areas of the brain, the globus pallidus and the thalamus. He had to close the artery off immediately, because of severe bleeding, and stop the operation to determine the effects of the accident.

When the patient awoke from anesthesia, the tremor and rigidity of Parkinson's disease had disappeared, without paralysis or other effect on motor functions.

After testing the new procedure's anatomical and surgical details on several baboons, Cooper repeated the surgery on fifty Parkinson's patients. One of those patients had, in addition to the shaking palsy, a dystonic deformity of his left hand. For the previous sixteen years his wrist had been permanently bent downward with the fingers painfully stretched toward the arm. Such a "fixed" deformity had never before been reversed. But after surgery the patient walked for the first time in ten years, and the dystonic hand became flexible and relaxed.

Cooper's observation of this side benefit was to lead, later on, to another breakthrough procedure to relieve the symptoms of a crippling hereditary disease called dystonia musculorum deformans.

Meanwhile, the surgeon kept refining his techniques, because he considered the operation on the tiny artery in the brain too risky and unpredictable: because the vessel nourishes slightly different portions of the brain in each individual, there was no telling what its effects might be. Cooper devised operations aimed at specific cerebral structures that he believed were the key to involuntary-movement disorders. His research led him to the thalamus, deep in the center of the brain. Using various chemicals, such as absolute alcohol, to make lesions in the thalamus itself, he improved the predictability of his results:

> Then one Christmas I received a gift of one of those little carbon dioxide wine-bottle openers. I was playing with it, and the carbon dioxide was cooling my hand, and I was thinking how much the device looked like a brain cannula (a probelike instrument). I got the idea of developing an instrument that would be a cannula, insulated on the sides with a cooling tip that could be put into different parts of the brain.

The bottle-opening gadget thus helped to open up a whole new field of surgical technique, which now has been used not only for brain procedures but also in operations ranging from eye surgery to hemorrhoid removal. It is called cryosurgery.

Cooper's deep-brain surgery for involuntary-movement disorders necessitated still another radical departure: the patient has to be awake during the operation. Before freezing and destroying part of the brain, Cooper cools the area in question. If the patient shows a relief of symptoms—in Parkinsonism the tremor stops the instant the appropriate area of the brain is cooled—without any side effects, the cryoprobe's temperature is lowered enough to kill the tissue. If the patient was anesthetized, however, that test could not be performed.

Today, cryothalamectomy for Parkinsonism is rarely performed because of the discovery, several years ago, of the beneficial effects of the drug L-Dopa. Before its successes were published, Cooper had learned about the L-Dopa work of Dr. George Cotzias of Brookhaven National Laboratory in New York. "I was so impressed by the effects [of L-Dopa] that I put an immediate moratorium on surgery for Parkinson's disease and canceled seven hundred operations." (Those seven hundred patients, and others, participated in approved clinical trials of L-Dopa at St. Barnabas.)

"The only Parkinson's patients we operate on now are those who have had good L-Dopa therapy in very competent hands and whose tremors haven't responded," Cooper says.

Today at St. Barnabas, where the cryothalamectomy operation for Parkinsonism was pioneered, and where up to 1,000 patients a year were once operated on, only a few such procedures are performed each month. Adds Cooper, "After having been an evangelist for this type of surgery for many years, I find that almost every other center is now doing more of it than we are." The irony of this point is not lost on Cooper, who remembers well the scorn many of those same physicians and centers once heaped on his discovery.

In *The New York Times Book Review* Lord C. P. Snow recently wrote that Cooper is "one of the most remarkable men alive. . . . He is regarded with intense respect, and something much warmer than that, by his English colleagues. They have told me that he attracts some envy, presumably because he appears to have all the gifts that a man might conceivably wish for."

At times Cooper's treatment of Parkinsonism was questioned because certain surgeons could not reproduce his results. Some doctors simply refused to believe that the disease could be reversed without paralyzing the patient. "Surgeons used to come here," Cooper recalls, "and watch us for a day or a couple of days and then go home and do the surgery. Some of them insisted on putting their patients to sleep during the surgery. But you just can't tell if you are putting the lesions in the right place unless the patient is awake and you can see his response."

A look back at the thousands of patients who received cryosurgery for Parkinsonism at St. Barnabas shows a mortality rate of less than 1.5 percent and lasting relief from tremor and rigidity in some 90 percent of good-risk patients. In poor-risk patients the success rate is about 60 percent. However, those who were not helped by his surgery are no worse off now than before.

I once watched a dramatic operation in which Cooper halted the tremors of an L-Dopa-resistant Parkinson's-disease patient. Afterward I told him his results were "miraculous." "No miracle," the neurosurgeon explained. "We doctors are only human. We do our best. But no miracles."

Some have questioned the propriety of Cooper's occasionally subjecting patients to radical procedures that have not first been perfected in experiments on animals. One reason for doing so is that there are no suitable animal "models" for many of the conditions being studied.

"We're talking about a patient," explains Cooper, "who has been sick not just for a week but for years and who is totally incapacitated, suffering both physically and mentally and willing to try anything. So I think the sole criterion should be the therapy of that patient."

In his recently published book, *The Victim Is Always the Same,* Cooper describes his own ethical-moral wrestling before he decided to operate on his first dystonic patient, an eleven-year-old girl. "How does one decide to place

167

for the first time an instrument deep in a child's brain and destroy part of it? It's not just a question of overcoming the technical difficulties, which can always be worked out in the laboratory. It's a more profound moral question than that, because only human beings have this disease."

Near the end of 1953 Cooper became the first physician to reverse the symptoms of dystonia. Now, with hundreds of cases behind him, his results can only be called dramatic. Seventy-seven percent of Cooper's patients have shown long-term reversal of symptoms, without sensory, motor, or intellectual impairment. In the rest of the cases, either surgery failed to reverse symptoms or they later reappeared. The mortality rate has been 2.7 percent. And although Cooper won't use the word *cure*, many of his patients have been symptom-free for ten years or more.

A few months ago I saw what dystonia does to a human being. While I was making rounds with Cooper one weekday, we saw a skinny, battered girl, twisted grotesquely in her hospital bed. Flailing her arms and legs, she moved about convulsively, banging her head and limbs on the metal sides of the bed.

The tearful mother explained that the disease had begun several years earlier, with small muscular distortions of the child's foot and leg. Doctors referred both the woman and child for psychiatric help, for they could find no physical basis for the disease. Psychotherapy did not help, and the disease progressed.

When the disease was finally diagnosed as dystonia, doctors told the woman it was hopeless. Hopeless— even though since 1953 Cooper's results had been widely known and published both in medical journals and in the lay press. Unfortunately, many doctors apparently chose to ignore the promise of Cooper's work. Then the child's mother wrote a plea for help to a medical newspaper, and it was published among the letters to the editor: "Can anybody help my child? She has dystonia."

Of the thousands of physicians who read the publication, none replied. But one, who had had a dystonic patient treated successfully by Cooper years before, passed the appeal along to that child's mother. Knowing personally the horrors of the disease, she wrote the woman about Cooper and his success with her own child, and told her, "Don't believe those who say his operation doesn't work."

From her home in the mountains of Pennsylvania, the mother brought the child to New York. Somehow, though, she first went not to St. Barnabas but to one of the city's other renowned medical centers. The chief of neurology there told the woman that nothing could be done for her child.

"What about Dr. Cooper?" the woman asked.

"His operation doesn't work," said the doctor.

Recalling the experienced mother's warning, the woman carried her child out the door—for she could no longer walk unassisted—and went to St. Barnabas.

And now she stood at the girl's bedside, weeping over the pitiful creature that was her daughter. The green-clad neurosurgeon could only shake his head grimly. He had lived it all too many times before. Within days the girl was operated on. Having learned that cerebellar stimulation can also relieve dystonic deformities, Cooper implanted a stimulator in her head.

I'm sorry to say, however, that I cannot report on the success or failure of that case. Only days after the surgery, just as the gradual cumulative effect of the stimulation had begun, the mother came to Cooper and insisted on taking her child home: "I had a dream that the girl will die no matter what we do." Cooper spent a day pleading with the woman to leave the child at the hospital. But his efforts were to no avail. The mother rescinded her permission for medical treatment, a decision legally within her rights as a parent, and took her child home.

The entire area of consent to treatment by the patient, or by the patient's guardian, is a crucial one. It takes on even greater significance when innovative procedures are involved. Cooper explains that a sick patient can never give a true "informed consent" to treatment. "The patient is never free, because he is imprisoned by his disease."

Some critics say that more carefully controlled operations on human beings must be undertaken before such procedures as the brain-pacemaker implantation can be considered effective. They have suggested double-blind testing in which, for example, half the patients would receive working stimulators and the other half would get "dummies." That approach is similar to using sugar pills in drug-efficacy studies. Cooper asks:

> What kind of controlled experiment can you do with these patients? You have to be honest with yourself and admit that you're working in a human situation and every case is different. In a drug study you can do a double-blind study. But you can't do that with the cerebellar stimulation. You can't open their heads and pretend to stimulate them.
>
> Anytime you put a patient to sleep (stimulator-implant patients, unlike cryothalamectomy patients, must be put to sleep because of the nature of the surgery), you risk his life. Who could do that in good conscience and then not even try to help them?

It's all a question of the surgeon's motives. Does he want to help people, or does he want to make discoveries that will embellish his own record? If the latter were the case with Cooper, as some have indeed charged, the surgeon would have left the small hospital in the Bronx years ago for greener pastures. (Cooper, incidentally, has worked essentially without government research grants over the last two decades. He plows 20 percent of his income back into his research, and St. Barnabas itself has contributed some $2 million in free patient care.)

"I'm convinced," Cooper says, "that motivation is an impossible thing to define. One thing that drives me is seeing someone who is sick and nobody else can help."

But what of the responsibility? "It's standard to operate for brain tumors, and everyone knows that when you operate for a brain tumor, the patient may die. But if you're going to operate on something that's never been operated on before, your responsibility multiplies a thousand times. And if you're the type of person who identifies with the patient, you are agonized."

At a recent meeting of the American Neurological Association, Dr. William Sweet, professor of neurosurgery at Harvard Medical School, praised Cooper's pioneering work with the brain stimulator. But he added that it would have been a tough job to get any hospital research committee to approve such an original piece of work.

"That's a valid criticism," says Cooper. "One of the things you have to start with, though, is that when you're dealing with humans, whatever you come up with is going to be imperfect and some of it will have to be judged after the fact. When you present people with so many things that are new, and some of them can't really be understood, you threaten their whole world."

He adds, however, "If I had operated on ten patients and they all had died, no matter how responsible I had been, then it would have been wrong. You have the ultimate responsibility to yourself to be right. And if you aren't, you must find it out quickly."

In the brain-pacemaker work Cooper has not been wrong. "Wayne A.," the first epileptic who received the system, has been essentially seizure-free for more than a year after his operation.

For the four previous years, however, Wayne A. had

been incapacitated by intractable epilepsy, apparently caused by a blow on the head from a baseball bat. He had full-blown seizures between one and five times a day and had bouts of nervousness and nausea another ten or fifteen times daily. These symptoms, plus a constant drowsiness caused by heavy but ineffective doses of anticonvulsive drugs, forced Wayne to drop out of college.

Today, Wayne's medication has been cut to less than a fifth of its previous level. Since surgery he has had several seizures, but all of them were linked to equipment malfunctions. Once it was discovered that a wire leading to the power source was broken, and Wayne admits that at other times, "I let my battery go dead."

It was before the turn of the century that British physiologist Sir Charles Sherrington found that stimulation of the anterior lobe of the cerebellum could ease decerebrate rigidity in cats. Fifty years later, young Cooper, then a fellow in neurosurgery at the Mayo Clinic, read a report on the work of Italian physiologist Giuseppe Moruzzi. The report said Moruzzi had found that electrical stimulation of the cerebellum could inhibit or facilitate motion, depending on the frequency used.

"I made a note in the book," Cooper recalls, "that chronic stimulation of the cerebellum in humans should relieve spastic states. I tried to work out the technology then but couldn't. Later my other work kept me too busy."

About two years ago, Cooper came across his earlier notation while he was preparing a lecture for medical students. "By then I had more time for reflection, and new stimulators were available. So I began working on chronic stimulation of the cerebellum." Before he began working with the stimulator, the neurosurgeon had considered retiring to write books. But now, he says, "We're just beginning what will be at least a five- or ten-year study. I'm sure that a number of our colleagues elsewhere will try out techniques so that many aspects will be studied. . . . This is an early phase of the work, and it has all the unknowns of any new work."

So Dr. Irving Cooper will continue his two pressing love affairs—with the human brain itself and with the patients for whom he feels so deeply.

Meanwhile, because of his pioneering success in controlling involuntary-movement disorders, a mechanic is returned to his tools, a doctor to his practice, a magician to his tricks. A lovely young girl who not so very long ago was grotesquely uncoordinated is now able to dance at her senior prom.

PART THREE

———— ● ————

The Spectrum
of Psychotherapy

Introduction
•
by Albert Rosenfeld

When, in the year 1793, an enlightened and humane physician named Philippe Pinel was put in charge of the infamous French mental hospital at La Bicêtre—a hellhole by any description—he created a sensation by freeing the vermin-infested inmates from their chains. Even in revolutionary France, so customary was the barbarous custodianship of the insane that Pinel was himself called mad for "freeing the beasts." But he was convinced that fresh air and freedom of movement were more curative than shackles and dungeons, and he was proved correct.

Though we still refer to our mental hospitals—which do, of course, leave much to be desired—as "snake pits," we can scarcely comprehend the unspeakable cruelties that were piously visited upon hundreds of thousands of wretched human beings in these institutions over the centuries. Their "treatment," which frequently included outright torture, was sanctioned by a book of horrors called *Malleus Maleficarum* ("Hammer to be Used Against Witches"), which was compiled by two scholarly monks toward the close of the fifteenth century. This studious

177

work "proved" that anyone afflicted with what we now think of as mental illness was possessed by demons and witches.

Pinel's courageous humanitarianism, as revolutionary as anything that occurred during the French Revolution, was a milestone in psychiatric history. It was, of course, a long, hard road from Pinel to Freud—and, though a much shorter time has elapsed, another long, hard road from Freud to us.

The period that we so recently referred to as "post-war"—the years immediately following World War II—is already ancient history from a psychiatric standpoint. In those olden days we had finally begun to believe that we knew and understood where we were, psychiatrically speaking. True, there did exist the more cursory and generally not very useful kinds of therapy offered in mental hospitals for really *crazy* people. So there was still the snake pit, but there was also the couch. Mainly, there was the couch.

Psychoanalysis held a special fascination for novelists, playwrights, and moviemakers, who helped popularize the analyst until almost all literate citizens could mouth terms like *id, libido, superego, sublimation, Oedipus complex,* and *phallic symbol.* Moreover, Freudianism gained almost undisputed ascendancy in academia. In their monumental work *The History of Psychiatry,* published in 1966, Drs. Franz G. Alexander and Sheldon T. Selesnick were able to exult over psychiatry's finally coming into its own as a full-fledged medical science. Giving the psychoanalytic movement much of the credit, they wrote: "Psychiatry has come of age. On the strength of substantial achievements, it has ceased being medicine's neglected step-child and has become one of the most prominent fields in medicine." Moreover, they felt that "civilization may have entered an age of psychiatry," and they applauded our new national awareness of the central importance of mental illness.

Yet, within a decade, the controversial American psychiatrist Dr. Thomas Szasz was making inroads in public awareness with his assertion that mental illness was merely a myth we had invented, and Dr. E. Fuller Torrey was saying flatly: "Psychiatry is dying." He allowed that this claim did seem ironic "in view of the fact that more people than ever are going to more psychiatrists than ever." Others claimed that psychiatry was neither a medical discipline nor a science. And there arose the influential school of Dr. R. D. Laing, which held, among a number of other suggestions, that a "disease" such as schizophrenia should perhaps not be cured at all. Laing proposed instead that the schizophrenic should be taken by the hand and permitted to go all the way with his illness—which was perhaps more sane than our sanity. The Esalen Institute held learned seminars on the uses of psychotic experiences. All these conflicting claims threw the public into great confusion.

Compounding this confusion was the bursting forth of new therapies. Suddenly, between the snake pit and the couch a diversity of options existed. "Breaking loose from the bonds of tradition," writes Dr. Harold Greenwald in *Active Psychotherapy,* "psychotherapy has recently undergone such a vast proliferation that it is almost impossible for even the most nimble of researchers in the field to keep up with the almost infinite variety of new approaches and new techniques." If even the experts in the field can't keep up, what can poor laypeople do? Bombarded on all sides by everything from "primal screams" to "I'm OK, You're OK" therapies, how does one sort out all the input? How do you separate the signals from the noise; how do you evaluate which, if any, of the new therapies make any sense—and where, meanwhile, has Freud gone?

The purpose of this section is to help sort out some of these confusions, to separate the signals from the noise. Dr. Morris Parloff, who keeps track of these trends for the National Institute of Mental Health, takes us on a quick tour of the new psychotherapies. Dr. Jarl Dyrud of the University of Chicago tells us where he thinks psychoanalysis now fits into the revised picture. And Dr. Seymour Kety of Harvard explains the importance of our new awareness of the biological aspects of mental illness and its psychopharmacological implications. Shorter articles treat such subjects as preventive psychiatry, depression, nutritional aspects of mental illness, and the special psychiatric problems of the disadvantaged.

We do not pretend to have cleared up all confusions, of course. As Dr. Joel Elkes of Johns Hopkins, a pioneer psychopharmacologist and psychiatrist, likes to say about psychotherapy, "If you understand the situation, you are not fully informed."

The Psychotherapy Marketplace

by Morris B. Parloff

There is nothing absolute about the aims of psychotherapy. They are, rather, tied closely to current standards of well-being and social effectiveness. In the past, these social standards seemed relatively fixed and stable. Today, however, our society changes its standards with ever-increasing speed, while the sciences keep fashioning new mirrors to reflect the new images of man. As a result, innumerable images are now simultaneously extant; which image we see depends on where we look.

At the same time, we make increasing demands on psychotherapy. In the past, religion and science were the main ways of achieving our aspirations. More recently, to the consternation of some and the satisfaction of others, the license for ensuring our well-being has apparently been transferred to psychotherapy.

The boundaries of the treatment, never firm, have become increasingly ambiguous and provisional; in fact, they now seem to be infinitely expansible. Within the

Dr. Morris B. Parloff, a clinical psychologist, is the chief of the Psychotherapy and Behavioral Intervention Section, Clinical Research Branch, National Institute of Mental Health.

past decade the role of the psychotherapist has been greatly extended. Not only is he expected to help the patient achieve relief from psychologically induced discomfort and social ineffectuality—that is, to treat "mental disorders"—he is also expected to help the client achieve positive mental health, a state presumably defined by the extent to which the patient experiences "self-actualization," growth, even spiritual oneness with the universe. Thus, some therapists have moved away from the earlier aim of "head shrinking" to the loftier goal of "mind expanding."

The range of problems brought to the psychotherapist has broadened to include not only the major mental disorders—the psychoses and neuroses—but also the celebrated problems of alienation and the meaninglessness of life. The conception of "pathology"—that is, what needs changing—has been modified. Where formerly the internal and unconscious conflicts of the *individual* were treated, the targets of change now encompass the interpersonal relationship, the family system, and, more recently, even society and its institutions.

Credentials for practicing psychotherapy have been broadened and, by some standards, lowered. What was initially almost the exclusive domain of the medical profession—of the psychoanalyst and psychiatrist—has slowly been opened up to include the related professions of clinical psychology, psychiatric social work, and psychiatric nursing. Among those more recently invited to provide some psychiatric services are the "paraprofessional," the nonprofessional, and even the former patient. The belief that "it takes (a former) one to treat one" has gained popularity, particularly in the treatment of drug abusers, alcoholics, criminals, and delinquents.

The number of "therapeutic techniques" also continues to grow. More than 130 different approaches are now being purveyed in the marketplace of psychosocial therapies.

New schools emerge constantly, heralded by claims that they provide better treatment, amelioration, or management of the problems and neuroses of the day. No school has ever withdrawn from the field for failure to live up to its claims, and as a consequence all continue to coexist. This remarkable state of affairs is explained in part by the fact that each school seems to be striving for different goals—goals reflecting different views of the "nature of man" and his potential. All approaches to treatment are sustained by their appeals to different constituencies in our pluralistic society.

By way of general introduction, I shall briefly review the four self-proclaimed major schools of psychotherapy. Then I will describe several other forms of treatment that are difficult to categorize but that currently also enjoy special popularity.

The four major schools of therapy are (1) analytically oriented therapy, (2) behavior therapy, (3) humanistic therapy, and (4) transpersonal therapy.

ANALYTICALLY ORIENTED THERAPY

The analytic (or psychodynamic, or depth) forms of therapy have evolved in a more or less direct line from classical psychoanalysis. While still flourishing, and perhaps the most frequently encountered form of treatment, this school appears—like unemployment and inflation—to be growing at a declining rate.

These psychodynamic therapies assume that people have innate and acquired drives that conflict with both the "external" requirements of society and the "internal" needs and "internalized" standards of the individual. Unacceptable drives are forced out of the conscious awareness—that is, repressed—but they continue, unconsciously or subconsciously, to press for expression.

A person's normal development may be interrupted by early-life experiences that either do not satisfy innate drives sufficiently or gratify them excessively. In either event, the child's development may be blocked. The emotions and fantasies derived from these unacceptable drives may be allowed partial expression in a disguised and compromised form. In some instances these emotions are "sublimated" into creative, socially beneficial channels. In other cases they "surface" as undesirable physical symptoms, or as socially unacceptable character traits and behavior patterns. The psychodynamic approach postulates that socialization is required in order for the person to become "human."

Psychoanalytic treatment tries to unravel internal problems by bringing the unconscious neurotic conflicts into the patient's consciousness. The direct target of treatment is not the patient's *symptoms,* but rather the forces that are believed to generate these symptoms.

The formula for bringing this repressed material squarely into the patient's awareness is: clarify, confront, interpret. Understanding and insight of this kind are presumed to be in themselves "curative," provided that they evoke emotional experiences of a compelling nature.

Typically, psychoanalytic approaches involve analysis of the relationship that the patient attempts to establish with the therapist. This relationship is presumed to mirror the patient's unresolved pathological childhood conflicts.

More recently, the analytically oriented therapist has begun taking into account the social and cultural context in which the patient lives. The classical treatment setting, restricted to patient-therapist pairs, has been widened to permit treatment in groups as well. Some psychodynamic therapies have moved from long-term to brief, time-limited courses of treatment. Though many of the classic procedures have been revised and relaxed, the basic assumption that dynamic forces underlie symptomatic behavior remains unchanged.

184

BEHAVIOR THERAPY

Most behavior therapy derives from laboratory studies of learning processes. The therapist does not postulate the existence of any disease, aberrant personality development, or internal underlying conflict. The problem is defined in terms of specific behavior that the patient or society considers to be maladaptive. The aim of treatment is to change behavior—to change, specifically, its frequency, intensity, and appropriateness.

The behavior therapist does not consider maladaptive forms of behavior evidence of "pathology" but rather as ways in which people have learned to interact with their environment. He believes that behavior disorders develop according to the same principles of learning evident in so-called normal learning.

Behavioral treatment begins with detailed study of the events that precede and follow occurrences of a particular behavior problem—phobic avoidances, compulsions, temper tantrums, sexual dysfunctions, and so on.

One major form of behavior therapy consists in changing environmental conditions that stimulate or maintain the unwanted behavior; this therapeutic technique is known as "operant conditioning." Behavior therapy now includes a broad spectrum of techniques, known by such names as systematic desensitization, assertiveness training, aversive conditioning, token economy, and modeling. These procedures are offered by psychologists, psychiatrists, educators, social workers, speech therapists, and others concerned with modifying behavior.

The procedure popularly labeled "biofeedback" is used as a potential treatment for a variety of psychosomatic disorders, such as headaches, insomnia, high blood pressure, asthma, circulatory problems, and backache. The primary principle in biofeedback (see "Biofeedback: An Exercise in 'Self-Control'" by Barbara Brown on page 34) is that if someone is provided with

185

information about certain changes occurring in his body, that person can "learn" to: (1) increase awareness of his or her bodily processes, and (2) bring these processes under conscious control. This control should then permit the patient to change the autonomic processes in a more benign or healthful direction. Awareness of events within the body is achieved by means of monitoring instruments, which detect the relevant internal physiological change, amplify it, and translate it into a visual or auditory display.

HUMANISTIC THERAPY

This umbrella term shelters a wide range of therapies and techniques. Perhaps the most important factor uniting them is their strong reaction against what they view as limited conceptions of human nature offered by the analytic and behavioristic therapies.

Humanists postulate that man is driven by an overarching need for self-actualization. Man's needs are, they assert, "higher" than simply mindless pleasure-seeking or avoidance of pain. Goodness, truth, beauty, justice, and order are not to be explained away as by-products of man's efforts to sublimate, divert, or block the direct expression of the baser drives that lurk within—an explanation sometimes attributed to analytically oriented therapy. Humanists believe that the failure to express and to realize the potential of higher human needs, motives, and capacities is the cause of emotional distress.

The goals of humanistic therapy are self-actualization and the enrichment and fuller enjoyment of life, not the cure of "disease" or "disorders." To realize your potential, you must develop increasing sensitivity to your own —and others'—feelings. Such heightened awareness will help establish warm relationships and improve your ability to perceive, intuit, sense, create, fantasize, and imagine.

The humanists stress that the only reality that merits

concern is one's own emotional experience—in contrast to what they view as the unwarranted faith that other therapists have placed in thought, insight, and understanding.

The analytic view holds that man's impulses must be frustrated and redirected in order that he be more fully human. But humanists argue that direct gratification of needs is ennobling and good.

Humanists such as the late Abraham Maslow hold that each individual has a biological essence, or self, that he must discover and develop, but that external influences are more powerful than biologically given characteristics and may distort or block our personal awareness and development.

The panoply of self-actualizing techniques ranges from nondirective counseling and Gestalt therapy to the multiple and ever-evolving variants of "growth" groups: the encounter group, the T-group, sensory-awareness training, and so on.

TRANSPERSONAL THERAPY

Unlike the humanists, the transpersonalists are not content with the aim of integrating one's energies and expanding the awareness of oneself as an entity separate from the rest of the universe. Instead, the transpersonalists' goal is to help the individual transcend the limits of ordinary waking consciousness and to become at one with the universe. The various levels and dimensions of awareness are as follows: "intuitive" states, in which vague, fleeting experiences of transsensory perception begin to enter waking awareness; the "psychical," in which the individual transcends sensory awareness and experiences integration with humanity; and the "mystical," representing a union of enlightenment in which the self transcends duality and merges with "all there is." Finally, there may be yet a further level of potential development—personal/transpersonal integrative—in which all dimensions are experienced simultaneously.

Transpersonalists do not share an organized theory or a clearly defined set of concepts, but, like the humanists, they assume that we all have large pools of untapped abilities, along with a drive toward spiritual growth.

One may achieve these levels by means of various techniques, including Arica training, the Gurdjieff method, Zen, psychosynthesis, Yoga, Sufism, Buddhism, and transcendental meditation.

Three transpersonal approaches have achieved considerable popularity: psychosynthesis, Arica training, and transcendental meditation.

Psychosynthesis was developed by a Florentine psychiatrist, Roberto Assagioli. As a form of therapy, it tries to help people develop "the will" as a constructive force guiding all psychological functions—emotion-feeling, imagination, impulse-desire, thought, and intuition. Treatment aims at enabling the patient to achieve harmony within himself and with the world as a path to attaining the higher self. It consists of techniques for training the will in order that one can master life and merge with "the universal will."

Arica training is an eclectic system, devised by Oscar Ichazo in Chile. It has incorporated many of the teachings of the Middle East and the Orient, including Yoga, Zen, Sufism, Cabala, and the martial arts. The branches of the Arica Institute now established in some major American cities stress these features: special diet, sensory awareness, energy-generating exercises, techniques for analysis in personality, interpersonal and group exercises, and various forms of meditation.

Transcendental meditation (TM), a variant of Raja Yoga, has become extraordinarily popular in the United States and Europe. This form of meditation has been adapted to the habits of Westerners and does not require special postures, forced concentration, lengthy or arduous training, or religious belief. Each person is assigned a mantra—a special incantation catch-phrase—which he is to keep secret and meditate on twice a day for about twenty minutes. This meditation helps people attain deep states of relaxation that are said to release creative energies. The advocates of TM hold that if a critical mass of 1 percent of the population in a given area meditates properly, the energies generated will benefit the rest of the population.

SPECIAL TREATMENT FORMS

Most techniques of psychotherapy can be included under one or another of these four rubrics—analytic, behavioral, humanistic, and transpersonal—but there remain a number of approaches that do not claim allegiance to any school and are not claimed by any. Some of these special approaches may be termed "pantheoretical"; others have evolved self-consciously "novel" techniques and procedures. The broad class of group psychotherapies and the many community-oriented therapies illustrate "pantheoretical" approaches; the "novel" therapies will be illustrated here by perhaps the best known—primal therapy.

"Group psychotherapy" does not represent any particular set of techniques or common philosophy of treatment. It refers to the *setting* in which the particular views and techniques of the analytic, behavioral, humanistic, and transpersonal schools have been implemented. In addition to having a knowledge of his own school, the practitioner of group psychotherapy must understand the dynamics and processes of small groups.

Of the many forms of group therapy, one of the best known is *transactional analysis* (TA), of *I'm OK, You're OK* fame. TA was developed by Eric Berne and represents an adaptation and extension of the psychodynamic orientation. The treatment attempts to identify covert gratifications—the "payoffs" of the "games" that people play with one another. The tasks of both the therapists and

189

the group patients include identifying the moment-to-moment ego states (parent, child, adult) that characterize each participant's interactions. A further step is to name the "game" that the individual is playing and, finally, to identify the "unconscious" life plan that the patient appears to have selected for himself during early childhood. The life plan involves the relatively enduring position of whether the self and others are "okay" or "not okay." The dynamics of change are believed to involve shifts of the "real self" from one ego state to another by an act of will.

Family therapy involves the collective treatment of members of the same family in a group by one or more psychotherapists. This approach treats not merely the individual but the family unit. The individual "patient" is viewed as but a symptom of a dysfunctional family system—a system that has produced and now maintains the problems manifested in a given family member.

The pantheoretical approaches include those therapies that extend the therapeutic focus to the community and society. The premise that environmental influences may interfere with a person's development has been taken up by a variety of therapists loosely associated with humanistic psychology. Perhaps the most extreme position is that taken by the group espousing *radical therapy,* which holds that society is responsible for most mental and emotional ills, and that, therefore, society rather than the patient is sick. People in psychological distress are considered oppressed rather than ill, and traditional psychotherapy is "part of the problem rather than part of the solution to human misery." The therapist attempts to help the patient recognize not merely his own problems but also the realities of his life situation and the role played by society in generating and perpetuating emotional problems.

Like radical therapy, *feminist therapy* believes that the root of emotional problems may be found in society rather than in the individual. Feminist therapy emphasizes that all psychotherapy must be freed of its traditional sex-role biases. Sexism is viewed as a major force impeding the "growth" of both men and women. This approach is not characterized by any particular techniques, but rather by a shared ideology. Consciousness-raising groups, too, which were initially politically motivated, have recently become oriented toward providing women with help for their personal problems.

Erhard Seminars Training, *est,* is a "philosophy/education process" and perhaps the fastest-growing, best-organized, most disciplined and most standardized form of "awareness training" currently available in the self-improvement industry. *est* is quite explicit in its disavowal of any psychotherapeutic intent and proposes instead to effect "transformation" rather than change. According to the proponents of *est,* individuals who undergo the experience can expect to be more fully alive, to feel complete, to enjoy radiant health, and to experience happiness, love, and self-expression. Since the aims of the psychotherapy client overlap many of these broad goals of self-enhancement, it can be assumed with certainty that many emotionally disturbed individuals will seek to explore this seemingly short route to a fuller and happier life.

The training program is characterized not only by its ineffable goals, but also by the rigor of its procedures and techniques. Approximately sixty hours of training are offered to groups of about 250 participants meeting over two successive weekends (Saturdays and Sundays). Each training day is usually interrupted only three times: twice for bathroom breaks and once for a meal. The procedures include a full statement of the conditions that the participants agree to accept. This contract authorizes the trainer to impose conditions of carefully planned privation, ridicule, humiliation, tedium and fatigue, a modicum of pain, considerable group pressure,

191

and group support and trainer approval. These conditions act to increase the accessibility of the participant to "experiencing one's own experience." The training also includes lengthy lectures, diatribes, and demonstrations by the trainer; responses (sharing) by the participants; and sets of "exercises" or "processes," which are aimed at enhancing relaxation skills, self-awareness, sense of worth, competence, and power. Successful completion of the training admits one to graduate status which offers eligibility to additional postgraduate training programs.

Primal therapy is viewed by its inventor, Arthur Janov, as unique in both its effects and its techniques, and as the "only cure of the neuroses." According to Janov, a neurosis occurs when the unexpressed physical and psychological pains experienced in childhood accumulate to the point where they are unbearable and can no longer simply be suppressed. The awareness of these feelings and needs is then "split off" when the child interprets the parents' behavior as meaning that they hate him. This formulation may occur at about the age of five or six and represents to Janov the "primal scene" that precipitates the neurosis.

In Janov's theory the pain of unmet needs is stored away somewhere in the brain and produces tension, which the patient may deal with by developing a variety of tension-relieving symptoms. Treatment requires the release and full expression of the underlying pain, by restoring physical access to the stored memories. Cure occurs only when each old painful feeling is linked to its origins. The living and reliving of the primal scene is accompanied by a "tower of terror" usually associated with screaming, violent thrashing about, pounding, and even convulsions. The screaming may go on for hours and may be repeated periodically over a period of many months as one event after another is recalled.

According to Janov, the cured individual should ideally have no psychological defenses, nor need any, since all pain and its associated tensions have been dispelled. The recovered patient thus becomes a "natural man," who is "nonindustrial, noncompulsive, and nondriving," and finds much less need for sex; women experience sexual interest no more than twice a month.

Even this truncated review of the major schools and techniques indicates the enormous complexity of any serious research effort that undertakes to compare the relative effectiveness of available therapies. Clearly, the basic conceptions differ as to who and what needs treating. It is not easy to prove that changes observed in patients or clients are due to the specific techniques and interventions. The therapist may wittingly or unwittingly provide the patient with experiences other than those assumed to be critical. It cannot be assumed that the same therapist will behave similarly with each of his patients—much less that different therapists espousing the same theory will behave similarly with all patients. The problems of research on the outcome of psychotherapy are further compounded by the concurrent impact of other events in the patient's life.

I shall report only the most consistent trends that emerge from a review of a large number of studies:
- Most forms of psychotherapy are effective with about two-thirds of their nonpsychotic patients.
- Treated patients show significantly more improvement in thought, mood, personality, and behavior than do comparable samples of untreated patients.
- Behavior modification appears to be particularly useful in some specific classes of phobias, some forms of compulsive or ritual behavior, and some sexual dysfunctions. Although behavior-therapy techniques appear to produce rapid improvement in the addictive disorders, such as alcoholism, drug abuse, obesity, and smoking, these changes usually are not maintained and relapse occurs in most cases.
- Biofeedback has been applied to tension head-

aches, migraines, hypertension, epilepsy, and some irregularities of heartbeat. The evidence, while encouraging, has not yet established such treatment as
being clinically significant.

• Meditation techniques of a wide variety all produce
comparable degrees of relaxation, with associated
physiological and metabolic changes. Currently,
"noncultist" adaptations of meditative procedures are
being applied with some success in the treatment of
anxiety, hypertension, and cardiac arrhythmias. Again,
findings must be viewed as tentative pending further
research.

• The criteria of "growth," "self-actualization," and
the attainment of transpersonal levels of consciousness remain ambiguous, and it is therefore difficult to
measure them objectively.

• Apparent differences in the relative effectiveness of
different psychotherapies gradually disappear with
time.

• Although most studies report that similar propor-
tions of patients benefit from all tested forms of therapy, the possibility remains open that different therapies may effect different kinds of changes.

All forms of psychotherapy tend to be reasonably useful for patients who are highly motivated, experience
acute discomfort, show a high degree of personality organization, are reasonably well educated, have had some
history of social success and recognition, are reflective,
and can experience and express emotion.

Jerome D. Frank has proposed that all therapies may
incorporate the same common (nonspecific) elements,
although in differing degrees: an emotionally charged
relationship with a helping person; a plausible explanation of the causes of distress; provision of some experiences of success; and use of the therapist's personal
qualities to strengthen the patient's expectation of help.

This statement in no way endorses tactlessness, insensitivity, or psychological assault. The therapist has no license to humiliate—or to thrill. A large-scale, careful study of participants who suffered psychological injury during encounter groups (led by acknowledged experts) revealed that the incidence of such casualties was disproportionately high among clients of so-called charismatic therapists, with their often aggressive, impatient, and challenging confrontation techniques.

No matter how specific the theory, no matter how clearly prescribed the techniques of a given therapy, treatment is far from standardized. Psychotherapy is mediated by the individual therapist and further modified by the nature of the interaction with the particular patient.

AFTERWORD:

Is Psychiatry a White-Middle-Class Invention?

—— • ——

by Ari Kiev

It has been charged that psychiatry is a white-middle-class invention, designed for use by white-middle-class practitioners for the benefit of white-middle-class patients. Though the charge is exaggerated, there is just enough truth in it to give us pause for careful thought.

As a peripatetic "transcultural" psychiatrist, I have had many opportunities over the past fifteen years to observe psychiatric practices throughout the world and to build a practice made up of patients from a diversity

---

Dr. Ari Kiev, author and lecturer, is a clinical associate professor of psychiatry at Cornell Medical School.

of types and cultures. I am constantly impressed by how special are the cultural contexts in which Americans are raised, what a striking difference these contexts can make in the kinds of emotional disturbances an individual may have, and which kinds of solutions may help him.

Although few psychiatrists are totally insensitive to these differences, doubtless many are only dimly aware of their own biases. I don't mean biases in the sense of being *anti* specific groups, but rather a tendency to let their own cultural biases and values influence their treatment methods and the goals they set for patients. It can be quite frustrating—or merely ludicrous if the patient has kept his sense of humor—for, say, a black man living in a high-crime area, or for a poverty-stricken reservation Indian, to be urged to attain his true human potential through self-actualization, or for an out-of-work depressed Appalachia resident to be told (by implication, usually) to snap out of it and pull himself together.

Many members of minority groups, particularly the poor, believe that they will receive little help or sympathy from an Establishment psychiatrist, and they may avoid seeking such help or do so reluctantly. An approach that fails to consider their particular preconceptions and cultural differences will result in rapid turnoff and dropout.

Some psychiatrists have little experience with poor people, simply because these patients can't afford to come see them in their private practices. Such patients may be seen in "charity" settings such as clinics or public mental hospitals, circumstances that can't help coloring the behavior and attitudes of both patients and psychiatrists. Disadvantaged groups have a higher-than-average representation in public mental hospitals simply because they *are* disadvantaged economically. They often have less family support and fewer adults on whom to model their behavior. They also have a higher rate of alcoholism and drug addiction. These afflictions do not respond very well to treatment in *any* group, but because of their preponderance in minority groups, it is all too easy to think of these patients as intractable *because* of their race or class.

Conversely, some enlightened psychiatrists may be so sensitive to cultural differences that they may forget that other cultural groups have absorbed at least part of—perhaps a large part of—American middle-class values, and that techniques that work with the general run of patients should not be totally abandoned. These doctors may forget, for instance, that hostility toward authority figures may be an important ingredient in a patient's problems whether he is a poor, middle-aged black man or a wealthy, teenage white boy. And either of the two persons may suffer from a lack of self-esteem or a lack of identity. Thus, the psychiatrist may see the same set of symptoms and really the same troubles in both persons —but *label* them differently (and sometimes mistakenly) purely because of the racial, ethnic, or cultural differences.

They may further begin to feel that they understand Italians or Jews or blacks or Indians or people with Spanish surnames—and to treat them as if they were all equally affected by the same cultural influences. But within any given culture, each individual is, well, an individual, and the cultural factors merely provide additional understanding as to what has shaped that individual.

On a recent morning, when I was running late because of an emergency, I noticed in my waiting room a backup of patients. Among them were an Irish nun and a bearded Hasidic rabbi, an affluent WASP businessman and a young black man who lived in one of Harlem's poorer neighborhoods. Now *there* was a diversity of cultures, right in that room; yet it would have been a mistake to assume that all these people needed to be treated entirely differently. The Irish nun, raised in a convent, and the Orthodox rabbi, who grew up in Hungary, had a number of problems in common. Both, for instance,

197

suffered from a marked obsession with perfectionism and from obsessive doubts about their own characters and abilities. The white corporation executive and the black ghetto youth both had an inclination to deny their symptoms and to minimize their need for treatment; and I knew that if I didn't exercise proper care (or even if I did!), there was a higher-than-average risk that they would drop out of therapy prematurely. My last two patients that morning, as it happened, were both teenage black girls from poor families—but oh, so different. One was from a rural Southern family; the other was a New York City native. One held rigidly puritanical views about sex, while the other was relaxed and easygoing in her sexual attitudes. They came from different universes in some respects; yet the fact that they both were black in today's United States did of course influence the development of both their personalities in a variety of ways.

In sum, then, one must be aware of both the similarities and the differences and always of the uniqueness of each individual. In the case of disadvantaged groups, the *culture of poverty* itself often exerts more influence than do their individual ethnic cultures.

There is no point or purpose in trying to convince intelligent women and men that their social and environmental conditions are fine when they're obviously bad, or in advising them to swallow their anger and indignation and compromise themselves. However, there is nearly always visible improvement when they understand, under sympathetic guidance, that not *all* their troubles are necessarily the result of outside circumstances, that—within given limits—they can gain some control and mastery over their own reactions and in turn their circumstances and personal futures.

Toward a Science
of the Passions
●
by Jarl Dyrud

The "impending death" of psychoanalysis is among its most time-honored traditions. At least since 1899, when Freud published his pioneering study of the mind, *The Interpretation of Dreams,* critics have been predicting (shedding no tears at the prospect) that the "talking cure" of Dr. Freud would be short-lived indeed. Yet, today psychoanalysis is still very much with us, having survived seventy-five years of putdowns from the scientific community and assaults from the adherents of assorted other forms of mental therapy. Though its *details* have been constantly modified, as is the case with any dynamic discipline, its *essence,* its central thrust and meaning, remains valid and vital.

How is it that psychoanalysis, with its roots deep in nineteenth-century individualism, manages to stay alive in the mid-seventies, when emphasis is all on the way people *behave* rather than on how they feel and think?

At least part of the answer comes through clearly in a recent *Psychological Reports* article by Arnold Lazarus,

Dr. Jarl Dyrud is associate chairman of the Department of Psychiatry at the University of Chicago.

titled "Where Do Behavioral Therapists Take Their Troubles?" Lazarus tells how he wanted to set up a meeting of leading behavioral therapists—that is, therapists with a strongly non-Freudian, nonpsychoanalytic outlook. But he found to his astonishment that most of them couldn't attend because of a conflict: the meeting fell on a day when they had appointments with their psychoanalysts!

Were these therapists hypocrites? Not really. The problems for which they were seeking psychoanalytic help were simply not *behavioral* in nature—that is, these therapists were perfectly able to get up in the morning, to do a day's work, and in general to behave perfectly normally. Their problems fell rather in that amorphous area claimed by analysis—the realm of meaning, of understanding, of trying to account for the "buzzing, booming" phenomena that churn about inside the human mind. This shifting inscape of private feelings is awkward territory for the conventional scientific mind, which shies away from anything that can't be weighed, measured, nicely categorized, and labeled. Thus, Freud's psychoanalytic method would seem to remain the only practical means of navigating through this stormy inner ocean of ideas and feelings.

True, the form of the problems addressed by psychoanalysis has somewhat changed. Earlier in this century, when Freud's ideas were still new, guilt and anxiety were the villains. Today, boredom and meaninglessness fester away inside us as we struggle for coherent meaning in our lives. But the essential *content* of psychoanalysis—its assumption that we can, with the analyst's aid, understand and alleviate our innermost conflicts—remains essentially what it was in Freud's day.

To be held within any reasonable limits, a status report on the totality of psychoanalysis must be highly subjective. I shall attempt the task by reflecting on the current health of (1) the revelation, (2) the method, and (3) the theory, including in the process some thoughts on the nontherapeutic applications of theory, the institutional arrangements, and future prospects.

The Revelation

The evolution of human awareness is not a smooth, steady continuum. Rather it proceeds in sudden, discontinuous steps, in which each move to a higher plane of awareness is achieved by revelation, by a new view of the human individual in his wholeness. Freud's articulation of the basic concepts of psychoanalysis is one of those revelatory steps in the evolution of consciousness. That revelation, to put it simply, provided us with the following concepts: *the dynamic unconsciousness* (our actions are determined by unknown forces); *transference* (we unwittingly carry attitudes born in old relationships into the new); and *consciousness as cure* (once we are made aware of what troubles us, it loses its hold on us). These concepts represent a real advance in our grasp of human possibilities. When a revelation such as Freud's initially occurs, it is radical and simple because it has been teased out for better visibility and in that sense has been, one might say, simplified or caricatured. We are probably neither so irrational as Freud—nor so rational as B. F. Skinner—would have us. As George Homans said about the nature of revelations, "To overcome the inertia of the intellect, a new statement must be an overstatement, and sometimes it is more important that it be interesting than that it be true." Any insight becomes more subtle and complex as it diffuses into a culture, but the new level of awareness remains. In that sense, psychoanalysis has *happened,* and there is no return to our lost innocence.

But why has there been so little progress following Freud's initial discoveries? It is puzzling how Freud's theoretical formulations, which he took pains to tell us were always incomplete and subject to revision, have shown such a strong tendency to get set in concrete.

The spin-offs from Freud of Jung, Adler, Ferenczi, and others—right down to the present day existential analyst *engagé*—do not really belong in this review because each in his own way represented not merely theoretical differences but an abandonment of the Freudian method itself, substituting a more active therapist contribution to the process. Within the movement itself a quiet center has remained. True, there has been a further elaboration of ego psychology, but on the whole we must admit there have been no more quantum leaps. This observation applies equally to the various schools of thought in psychoanalysis where the arguments seem more often based on personality clashes rather than on significant differences. It could be that our expectations have been geared to a false premise—that is, that psychoanalysis was a new discovery opening the twentieth century. If we were to look at psychoanalysis rather as the last statement of a nineteenth-century development, it might be easier to understand.

The actual evolutionary step in human awareness very likely began around 1800. As Karl Weintraub points out in *Critical Inquiry,* at about that time a radical change took place in man's self-consciousness, which was made evident by the sudden increase in autobiographical writing. Whereas all autobiographical writing prior to 1800 can be listed on two or three pages, a bibliography of nineteenth-century autobiographies comprises a weighty tome. This new ability to stand aside and look at oneself as an individual, to examine personal motives and experience in relation to surrounding events and individual encounters, may well have established the evolutionary context in which Freud was able to articulate the principles involved. It might be fairer to say that Freud transmitted an awareness of this subjective view of man, developed over an entire century, to the liberal intellectual culture of the twentieth century.

The Method

As a therapy, the psychoanalytic method of investigation is widely employed today. Free association as a method of gaining access to the symbolic process is a form of midwifery of meaning that works. I'm tempted to say that psychoanalysts sample the stream of thought much as scientists sample the bloodstream for indications of health or illness. But psychoanalysis as a *research* method has encountered both real and artificial difficulties. The real difficulties include such problems as how to gauge the accuracy of the analyst's *intuitive* responses to his patient, as opposed to the simpler task of demonstrating flaws in the patient's *logic*. The artificial difficulties lie in such areas as the therapist's reluctance to tape-record, videotape, or in any other way monitor the process—or to permit any third party to do so. This conflict between wanting psychoanalysis to be, on the one hand, a science among other sciences with "hard" data and, on the other, the art of saying the right thing at the right time without the contaminant of outside observation, is not easily resolved. The impasse stems in part from the nature of the practitioners, who are sophisticated in clinical method but naïve in research method, and in part from the intrinsic nature of the subject.

This urge to win scientific respectability has not been confined to psychoanalysis. All the twentieth-century social sciences have aspired to be "harder" sciences, in many instances following economist Frank Knight's humorous corollary to Lord Kelvin's dictum, "If you cannot measure it, your knowledge is meager and unsatisfactory." Knight added, "And if you can't measure it, measure it anyway."

Arbitrary definition of units to be counted has given economists headaches enough in their efforts to make explanations—to say nothing of predictions—in the area of human economic behavior. In psychology it has led to much counting of trivia, but, more important, it has led to discounting all that is human that cannot be counted. Meager and unsatisfactory though it may be, we need a science of human passions and possibilities. Considering that the psychoanalytic method is expensive and time-consuming, that training for the work is equally long and costly, and that formal *research* training is not a part of it, I think that most analysts have properly opted for the art of practice.

There has been much confusion about the way learning takes place in analysis. Accusations of "dogmatic Freudianism" imply a rigid adherence to a jargon that reduces the mystery and richness of an individual life to a formula. When such reductionism occurs, and it does, it might more appropriately be called "psychoanalytic behavior modification," because with it has gone the method as well as all elements of surprise and discovery. To be Freudian in outlook is for the analyst as well as the patient to feel a bit anxious before a session, because neither of them knows what is going to emerge. To maintain conviction in the face of uncertainty, the analyst has Freud's revelation and his method; he does not require any supportive dogma.

Searching for meaning, accounting for objects, events, and experiences in one's environment, has been with us ever since Adam named the animals, because naming is the beginning of language. One of man's most striking characteristics is that he is a pattern maker. He names not only natural objects but also thoughts, feelings, and relationships perceived in time or in space. He is perpetually organizing them into some sort of scheme that provides answers to questions growing out of his experience. This tendency to weave a seamless garment of meaning appears in the fantasies and fairy stories of children and in their ideas about where they came from, where they go when they die or go to sleep, and the like. In adults, it appears in, among other things, conspiratorial views of politics and history, delusional systems and compulsive rituals, the rationalizations that pass for explanations and understandings in everyday life, and even the best scientific theories and intellectual inventions. The test of these geometries of meaning does not lie in their truth but in their usefulness. They must be shared beliefs, at least to the extent that they permit one to live in one's community with a modicum of comfort and participation. In that sense, twentieth-century man still tends to exist like Evans-Pritchard's Azande people in Africa, "in whose web of belief every strand depends on every other strand, so that one cannot get out of its meshes because it is the only world he knows. The web is not an external structure in which he is enclosed. It is the texture of his thought, and he cannot think that his thought is wrong." Psychoanalysis provided a systematic way of penetrating that web and opening it up to the possibility of change as no other experience could. It provided a safe occasion for the suspension of belief so that one could see beyond the appearances and gain a larger view of the self. Thus, the psychoanalytic method has proved valid in practice even though it has never been—and perhaps cannot be—validated in terms of quantifiable scientific data.

THE THEORY

The same lack of precise scientific verifiability explains, in part, why psychoanalysis, as psychological theory, has had heavy going in spite of its broad clinical acceptance. Another source of difficulty is the usually ignored fact that psychoanalysis is not one theory but rather *two*—which are so intertwined as to cause inevitable confusion. The theory on which Freud worked the hardest is called metapsychology; this is a highly abstracted set of terms for things (processes and events) presumed to be going on in the mind—though, again, not provably so. Many of these terms (*cathexis, Eros, death instinct,* and the like) have become a minor part of the popular vocabulary, but they are too far removed from body language and feeling experience to carry much conviction. Metapsychology was supposed to provide a genuine scientific theory modeled on theories in the physical sciences that would be objective, rather than subjective, in character. Unfortunately, it was more a speculative neurophysiology, independent of the data of the psychoanalytic interview, than it was a psychology. It strove for the *how* of an impersonal process rather than the *why* of a slip of the tongue or a momentary forgetting. For a long time clinical inferences were taken as facts from which metapsychological theory could be abstracted. It is now more generally recognized that this network of inferences, even though closely linked with experiences in the consulting room, *is* theory. The second theory, which grows directly out of experience, seems to have less science about it, because it deals with man as a creature who has highly subjective intentions and strives after meaningful goals. This theory, strongly interpersonal in character, lives with language in that middle ground between mentalistic and behavioral. If we don't feel the need to prove that psychoanalysis is or is not a science, and are content instead to look, with the psychoanalyst, at the patient's strategies arising from his own attributions of meaning and intention, then we see that these purposes can be dealt with adequately without the need to translate them into another system.

Psychoanalytic inferences, generalizations, and clinical theory *do* have close links with feeling experience, but they need not be dogma. The terms are really shorthand symbols for referring to events in the dialogue of treatment. Expressions such as *repression, defense, return of the repressed, regression, the Oedipus complex, castration anxiety,* and, of course, *penis envy* (the current bane of radical feminists) have become American household words.

Taken out of context, treated as truths about human nature, they lose their value. For instance, castration anxiety really describes a shrinking genital sensation so well that it is difficult to remember that this adjective and noun are not literally appropriate but are simply a metaphor for a range of experiences in growing up. The analytic work involves the verbs and adverbs of what is and has been going on rather than mere labeling.

The issue is not to get down to the fundamental structures of the human mind but rather to find ways to help the patient revise idiosyncratic conceptions that are crippling him. Oscar Wilde commented that people who insist on probing deeply are really shallow because they pursue generalities. Those who pursue the shallower patterns of an individual life achieve true depth in comprehending another person. This is not to say that we learn nothing from experience. Over long periods of time, clinical observations can be accumulated and shared to form generalizations about common patterns of problems relevant to our culture and to our time. The psychoanalytic method does in that sense reveal a reality much as good literary criticism does, without excluding other realities. It enables the patient to explore and take into account more facets of his life and to see them in different perspectives in a relationship that supports his choosing to become a more whole and capable person.

Like Saul Bellow's Von Humboldt Fleisher, I feel the necessity of touching on everything in passing. A word must be said about the application of theory in non-therapeutic situations. Freud set the example for psychoanalytic biography and literary criticism. None of that came off too well, but it did illustrate that psychoanalytic literary detective work (psychohistory) can be fun. Erikson's *Young Man Luther* is a good example. It involves applying a disciplined and receptive imagination to the written record with occasionally brilliant new insights. What is critical is not that psychohistorical works exclude other interpretations, but that they enrich us by including more.

One of the problems of the diffusion of psychoanalysis into popular culture is that many purveyors of the ideology have no training in the method or any conception of it. Reading by itself apparently invites writers to use psychoanalytic terms as a tarot deck for the interpretation of history, literature, or the "root causes" of social problems. There is a reductionist quality to so many of these pseudoexplanations because there is no recognition that though this form of imaginative work may add a dimension, it does not replace prior dimensions of a problem. It is not "what is really going on." Just as we know by now that the ghetto does not in and of itself produce crime, and the suburbs do not promote mental health, we also know that psychoanalytic understanding is no substitute for objective data. Certainly those who see psychoanalytic ideology as a revolutionary political and social force for good, as so many of our public protagonists seem to, are often dismayed to find that the main offering of psychoanalysis is a slow and often painful stripping away of illusion. If one is strong enough, one can get through unpleasant discoveries to the somewhat stoic but satisfying philosophy that psychoanalytic theory represents. We must bear in mind that the only prescription for change put forward by Freud was the individual increase of satisfaction and efficiency that comes from the application of the psychoanalytic method.

RETROSPECT AND PROSPECT

Prior to World War II psychoanalysis was more of an intellectual movement than an institution. Talented, often-troubled people were drawn to practice it. Within the field of psychiatry it was a low-prestige, low-paying pursuit. But psychoanalysis had its own rewards of intellectual adventure and emotional satisfaction. Admission to training was based on interest and presented few obstacles. There were not only casualties but also a slowly increasing number of extremely able and gifted psychoanalysts. Following World War II—in this country in particular—psychoanalysis moved from a minority "family type" in-group to an institution of high prestige and intellectual domination of the field. For a time psychoanalysis dominated psychiatric training and captivated a generation of professional minds as the treatment that should if possible be made available to everyone. This of course flew in the face of psychological and economic realities. Psychoanalysis requires a patient who is healthy enough to tolerate the ambiguity of listening mostly to himself and is endowed with enough time and money to dedicate a number of years to the project. It became apparent that the majority of patients needed guidance, medication, or other more structured and focused methods of intervention for part if not all of their care. As a result, a variety of alternative therapies is available today, not all of them on the lunatic fringe. In many cases we now can look for a number of responsibly safe and less-time-consuming attempts to deal with human misery.

One of the products of that period of high prestige was a blurring of the psychoanalyst's role. Naturally, the field began to attract a broader spectrum of candidates for training, not all of whom felt particularly drawn to the work itself. Being a psychoanalyst became more significant than doing psychoanalysis. This change of focus worries an increasing number of analysts who are interested in exploring the opening in the web of belief rather than in trade-union issues. A few years ago the American Psychoanalytic Association conducted a study that demonstrated that a good percentage of the clinical time of psychoanalysts was spent in the role of seasoned clinician—doing consultation and referral work as well as brief and less intensive psychotherapy. I call them seasoned clinicians, because I think psychoanalysts are by and large a capable lot. The intensive scrutiny of themselves, their own motivations, combined with long supervised work with patients, does tend to make them perceptive. Perhaps their perceptiveness is not quite the same as that of Tolstoi's talented lady novelist, who could spend five minutes looking through the window of a barracks and know all she needed to know about soldiering, but they are able to make quick, intuitive judgments with less than complete information. This form of divination can certainly be done best by the best-trained person; it is of great value in individual, group, family, or pharmacotherapy; but it is no substitute for patiently teaching a patient to analyze himself, which is the goal of the method.

Where then is psychoanalysis today? In brief, the revelation is in good shape, the method suffers somewhat from neglect, the theories are in a healthy flux, and the institution is too comfortable to suit a growing number of its members. Encouragingly, these psychoanalysts do not accept splitting off as a solution to their discomfort. They want institutional change.

Psychoanalytic ideology has become a part of our contemporary web of belief. It is now the reference point not only for the new therapies that are action-oriented derivations of it but also for the behavior therapies originally proposed as alternatives to it. In this climate it seems likely that clinical psychoanalysis will survive, focusing its skeptical lens on literal acceptance of any ideology, including psychoanalytic ideology.

And Now,
Preventive Psychiatry

by Albert Rosenfeld

One of the most exciting and innovative areas in psychotherapy today is preventive psychiatry. It is a movement
that has spread rapidly, almost explosively, over the past
few years; even so, many communities throughout the
land still have not been touched by it. Symbolic of its
power for good is the work of one of the pathbreaking
institutions in this field—the Center for Preventive Psychiatry (CPP) in White Plains, New York, where Dr. Gilbert W. Kliman, author of *Psychological Emergencies of
Childhood,* directs a professional staff dedicated to head-
ing off emotional troubles before they are well begun.
Other preventive programs have arisen in various parts
of the country, but CPP remains unique in its across-the-
board concern with the entire range of preventive-
psychiatric services and its willingness (though its essential orientation is psychoanalytic) to draw on a varied
repertoire of psychiatric techniques. In the ten years of
CPP's existence, it has prevented thousands of personal
and family emotional disasters through the prompt and
knowledgeable application of what might be called "psychiatric first aid."

Though preventive psychiatry qualifies as a "new frontier," what it preaches is an old-fashioned, stitch-in-time philosophy: a little therapy now may save a lot of therapy later. In fact, in some circumstances, a little now may forestall events that would later be beyond repair. What preventive medicine represents for physiological illness, preventive psychiatry hopes to achieve for emotional troubles.

One major emphasis of preventive psychiatry, especially as practiced at CPP, is the early detection of children who are "at risk," psychiatrically speaking. Most troubled children, unless their behavior is too wildly aberrant to be ignored, are not identified as candidates for psychotherapy until well after they've started school. By then it is often too late to give them substantial help, and it takes much greater efforts to undo the damage even partially. By educating the community (Westchester County)—especially people in key positions, such as parents and nursery-school teachers—CPP has been able to rescue hundreds of children of *preschool age,* from infancy to six, the years most neglected both by agencies and by private therapists. Many of these children might otherwise have been declared autistic or hopelessly retarded (indeed, some had already been so declared) and would perhaps have required lifetime custodial care. Human tragedies that were considered inevitable, irretrievable, have now, in many cases, become preventable, thanks to new techniques worked out at CPP.

One example is the "Cornerstone method." Instead of a troubled child's being confronted with an analyst in his office on a one-to-one basis, a small group of such children go to the Cornerstone Nursery School at CPP. In the classroom they undergo the same kind of play and learning experiences as children do in other nursery schools—except that in this instance they do so under the watchful eye of an analyst and two teachers with special therapeutic training. In the classroom setting, in natural interactions with other children and teachers,

212

insights that might have taken months of patient therapy to draw out may often be attained much more quickly and may offer understanding of the troubles of more than one child at a time. Thus, the classroom has proved to be a marvelous multiplier and accelerator of therapeutic effectiveness.

But preventive psychiatry is for people of all ages and circumstances. The first-aid concept doesn't require that its clients (not *patients,* necessarily) suffer from a "mental illness." One of CPP's specialties is "crisis intervention," another psychiatric trend, and this busy department (the Situational Crisis Service) is directed by Ann Kliman. In this role she has recently been called upon to offer a truly pioneering type of service, psychological disaster-aid programs for entire communities: Corning, New York, after the flood; Xenia, Ohio, after the tornado. But she and her colleagues usually deal with troubled individuals and families.

In most places in the world, a situational crisis is not something that brings people in for psychiatric treatment. Ordinarily, these are situations you expect to manage yourself, perhaps with the help of friends and family —the kind that could happen to almost anyone (though perfectly sane and untroubled) at almost any time, and that are likely to occur to everyone at some time in life.

What, then, constitutes a situational crisis? A death in the family. A serious, chronic illness, especially of a parent. A home destroyed by fire. An automobile-accident injury. A lost job, especially if the period of unemployment lasts awhile. It could be something as routine as moving from one city to another or even from one house to another, depending on family circumstances and the ages of the children.

Around Westchester people are learning the importance of preventive psychiatry. Usually they are referred by doctors or clergymen. Often they come directly. In helping people through a crisis, the psychotherapist makes no attempt to *abolish* their troubles—that would be foolish and futile—but rather to help people *master* their troubles and come through them whole.

The therapy is as short-range as circumstances will allow. Some members of a family may need more help than others. An "average" case may require, say, two sessions a week for a period of several weeks. These may be held at CPP or at the client's home. People may be seen individually, in whole-family sessions, or both. Additional help may be drawn from anywhere: friends, relatives, clergymen, physicians, attorneys, teachers, community agencies. No two cases are quite alike. Everything depends on what happened, and under what circumstances.

Many situational crises cannot be expected to have a happy ending in the storybook sense. A tragedy is tragic, and a disaster is disastrous. There is no way CPP's preventive psychotherapists, with all their accumulated wisdom and experience, can bring back the dead father, the burned-down house, the ailing mother's health, the lost job. What they can do—with great success—is to escort the victims, chaperone them gently through the crisis, to ascertain that there *will* be an end to it, that it will be dealt with and finally put to rest. The preventive psychotherapists prevent the ending from being any more *un*happy than is absolutely necessary. They keep the tragedy from stretching out through troubled years, even through troubled lifetimes. And by providing fresh understanding and a sense of self-renewal, preventive psychotherapists sometimes confer upon the patients the gift of something very like a happy ending.

The Biochemical Roots
of Mental Illness
by Seymour S. Kety

Mental illness, although not a major cause of death, like cancer or heart disease, nevertheless ranks as one of our most serious national health problems. More than 10 million Americans will experience one or more episodes of serious mental illness, which may last for only a few weeks or even for many years, before they reach old age. The care of the mentally ill, inadequate as it often is, costs this nation considerably more than $5 billion annually—and less easily calculated is the larger human cost to the victims and their families.

For two mental illnesses that at one time rivaled schizophrenia in severity and extent—general paresis and pellagrous psychosis—biomedical research discovered the causes: an invasion of the brain by the spirochete of syphilis for one, and a dietary deficiency of nicotinic acid for the other. This made possible their effective treatment and prevention through purely biological processes. As a result, these disorders have practically disappeared in America; where they do occur, the cause is a

---

Dr. Seymour S. Kety, of Harvard University and the Massachusetts General Hospital, is a leading authority on the biological aspects of mental illness.

215

failure by society to utilize available scientific knowledge.

But schizophrenia and the so-called affective disorders (depression and manic-depressive psychosis) have remained with us, and their seriousness is matched by our ignorance regarding them. We do not yet know their causes or understand the processes through which they develop. Their treatment, which has improved dramatically through the use of recently discovered drugs, still leaves much to be desired. However, over the past two decades substantial indications have revealed that these serious mental illnesses have biochemical underpinnings, and powerful new techniques and concepts have been developed that make the search for these remedies more promising than it has ever been before.

The idea of a biochemical cause of insanity is not new. The Hippocratic physicians of ancient Greece argued against the prevailing attribution of insanity to supernatural causes:

> . . . and by the same organ [the brain] we become mad and delirious and fears and terrors assail us, some by night and some by day, and dreams and untimely wanderings and cares that are not suitable and ignorance of present circumstances, desuetude and unskillfulness. All these things we endure from the brain, when it is not healthy but is more hot, more cold, more moist, or more dry than natural, or when it suffers any other preternatural and unusual affliction.

The modern biochemical approach to mental illness can be traced to J. W. L. Thudichum, a physician and biochemist, who, nearly a hundred years ago, hypothesized that many forms of insanity were the result of toxic substances fermented within the body, just as the psychosis of alcohol was the result of a toxic substance fermented outside. Armed with the hypothesis, he received a ten-year research grant from the Privy Council in England. He did not go to the mental hospitals and examine the urine and blood of patients; instead he went to the abattoir to obtain cattle brain and spent the ten years studying the brain's normal composition. It is fortunate for us that he did that, because he laid the foundations of modern neurochemistry, from which will come whatever we learn about the abnormal chemistry of the brain. If Thudichum had been less wise and courageous, or if Parliament had insisted on "relevant" research, what contribution could he have made with the little knowledge that existed at that time? What chances would he have had to identify abnormalities in substances unknown in his day? He would have frittered away the public funds and wasted ten years in a premature and futile search.

Thudichum and the science of neurochemistry he founded were concerned at first with composition and chemical structure. In the normal brain a large number of substances were identified that were later found to be abnormal in a substantial variety of neurological disorders. Fifty years ago biochemistry began to trace the complex metabolism by which foodstuffs and oxygen are utilized and energy is made available. This understanding was eventually applied to the brain, where its dependence on glucose was discovered, and the oxygen utilized in various mental functions could be measured. Application of this knowledge to the states of sleep, coma, anesthesia, and senile dementia soon followed. But the major psychiatric problems (schizophrenia and manic-depressive psychosis and depression) remained unaffected. No known changes in chemical composition or structure account for these disorders; the brain uses just as much oxygen thinking irrationally as rationally.

Over the past twenty-five years there has been dramatic and unprecedented growth in the neurosciences and in our knowledge of the brain and behavior. One major new concept is that of the synapse, the highly specialized junction between one nerve cell and another through which information is carried. Electron microscopy, biophysics, biochemistry, and pharmacology have taught us a great deal about the synapse's structure and function. Most novel and far-reaching is the knowledge that chemical mediators called "neurotransmitters" carry the message over a small gap (the synaptic cleft) that lies between the termination of one nerve cell and the beginning of another. Because sensory processing, perception, the storage and retrieval of information, thought, feeling, and behavior all depend upon the operation of these chemical switches, this discovery elucidated the focal points at which chemical processes and substances, metabolic products, hormones, and drugs could modify these crucial aspects of mental state and behavior. If there are biochemical disturbances in mental illness, they would be expected to operate there, and drugs that ameliorate these illnesses should exert their influences at synapses.

There are hundreds of billions of synapses in the human brain, and they are organized in a marvelously systematic way along pathways that neuroanatomists are mapping. A growing list of neurotransmitters is being identified, and these are found to be associated with particular pathways, functions, and behavioral states. The class of substances known as catecholamines includes adrenalin, noradrenaline, and dopamine, first identified in the adrenal gland or in the peripheral sympathetic nervous system. Catecholamines are now known to be important neurotransmitters in the brain, where they appear to be involved in emotional states such as arousal, rage, fear, pleasure, motivation, and exhilaration. Serotonin, first discovered in the blood and the intestine, has also been identified as a neurotransmitter in the brain, where it seems to play a crucial role in sleep and wakefulness, in certain types of sexual activity, and perhaps in modulating, damping, and balancing a wide

218

range of synaptic activity that we are only beginning to understand. Acetylcholine, which is known to be the transmitter between nerve and muscle and is therefore crucial to every voluntary movement, has also been found to be involved in a very large fraction of brain synapses. There are other neurotransmitters, such as gamma amino butyric acid, certain amino acids and poly-peptides discovered more recently, and undoubtedly many that are as yet undiscovered. The importance of the concept of chemical neurotransmission and its im-plications for medicine and psychiatry was recognized by the Nobel Committee, which gave the award in 1970 to Julius Axelrod, Bernard Katz, and Ulf von Euler for their contributions to the understanding of acetylcholine and catecholamines as neurotransmitters.

Fundamental knowledge of the synapse and chemical neurotransmission has had important implications for the understanding and treatment of nervous and mental disease and represents an area of unusual promise for the future. At the same time that noradrenaline and serotonin were being identified in the brain, several drugs were discovered quite independently to exert im-portant effects on mood. The first of these was reserpine, which has been found to be useful in the treatment of hypertension. In a small percentage of patients, how-ever, reserpine produced a state of depression very much like that known to psychiatrists. At the same time, scientists at the National Institute of Health made the important discovery that reserpine causes the disappear-ance of serotonin and noradrenaline from the brain.

A few years later a new drug, iproniazid, was intro-duced and found to be highly effective in the treatment of tuberculosis. It caused excitement in some patients, however, and was supplanted by other drugs equally effective and without such side effects. What was a deleterious property of iproniazid in the treatment of tuberculosis, however, became the basis for an effective

219

treatment of depression. Iproniazid was found to block the enzyme monoamine oxidase (MAO), which is responsible for inactivating biogenic amines, including serotonin and the catecholamines, in the brain. Thus, iproniazid exerted an effect on these transmitters opposite to that of reserpine, permitting them to rise in concentration and activity and exert an antidepressant effect. A number of other MAO *inhibitors* were developed that were also effective in treating depression. Even more effective were a group of drugs, the tricyclic antidepressants such as imipramine and amitryptaline, which enhanced the synaptic actions of noradrenaline and serotonin by yet another mechanism.

Thus, depletion of these two neurotransmitters is associated in animals and man with depression, while the drugs that restore their levels and increase their synaptic activity are effective antidepressants.

It is a reasonable inference from the foregoing observations that clinical depression may be the result of an inadequacy of one or both of these neurotransmitters at particular synapses in the brain—and similarly that mania, the obverse of depression, may represent an *overactivity* of such a transmitter. Testing such hypotheses has engaged a number of research groups. There have been some interesting findings, e.g., that in certain types of depression and in mania there is in the urine a decrease or an increase respectively of a particular product of noradrenaline metabolism that appears to be derived largely from the brain. Others have found in cerebrospinal fluid evidence of a decrease in serotonin metabolism in the brain in patients suffering from manic or depressive psychosis. A very effective agent in the treatment of mania and the prophylaxis of manic-depressive illness is lithium, a relatively simple substance closely related to sodium, which plays a crucial role in synaptic function. The mechanism by which lithium produces its therapeutic and prophylactic action is as yet unknown, although recent observations suggest that it enhances the synthesis of serotonin.

Similarly, over the past two decades, newly acquired knowledge has begun to unravel the enigma called schizophrenia. This disorder or group of disorders (we may be dealing with a number of different diseases with a common symptomatology) is characterized by disturbances not only in mood but also in thinking and the normal association between mood and thinking. In the typical severe schizophrenic one sees bizarre behavior, disorders of thinking and speech, impoverishment of feeling, lack of motivation, anhedonia (an inability to experience pleasure), withdrawal from interaction with others, hallucinations, delusions, and educational, occupational, social, and marital disabilities. Such symptoms appear insidiously early in life and become critical in early adulthood. There are such drugs as mescaline, LSD, or dimethyltryptamine, which are capable of inducing hallucinations and some of the other symptoms of schizophrenia, and have, for some, suggested hypotheses about the nature of schizophrenia itself.

What most hallucinogenic drugs have in common is one or more methyl (CH_3) groups. It is, therefore, especially interesting that an enzyme has been found in body and brain tissues of animals and man that is capable of adding a methyl group to *normal* metabolites, thus converting them to hallucinogenic substances. To date, however, no such hallucinogenic substance has been clearly identified in schizophrenics. In 1950 a new drug was found to be more effective than any previous treatment in the relief of some of the major symptoms of schizophrenia. That discovery came about in an interesting and unexpected manner. Pharmacologists had been developing and studying drugs that blocked the actions of histamine, a substance manufactured within the body, which appears to play an important role in many forms of allergy. The antihistaminic drugs thus elaborated have been found to be very beneficial in the treatment of asthma and other types of allergic disorder. One of these drugs was found to combine both antihistaminic and sympatholytic properties—i.e., it also blocked the actions of the sympathetic nervous system.

Henri-Marie Laborit, a French anesthesiologist, was looking for a drug that had such properties as a means of preventing surgical shock, on the hypothesis that both histamine and sympathetic overactivity contributed to its development in surgical operations. He used this drug in preoperative medication, and, because he was a careful observer, he noted in his patients the occurrence of an unwanted and unsearched-for sedation, a kind of sedation different from that which occurs with the barbiturates—a "euphoric quietude." He felt that such a property might be helpful in treating disturbed patients and suggested that to psychiatrists. That drug was the immediate forerunner of chlorpromazine, which revolutionized the treatment of schizophrenia. Chlorpromazine was tried in Paris and very quickly elsewhere in Europe, England, Canada, and the United States. It became the first of a series of "major tranquilizers" or "antipsychotic" drugs, so named because of their rather specific ability to terminate or ameliorate the psychotic manifestations of schizophrenia, especially the bizarre behavior and thinking, the delusions and hallucinations.

But chlorpromazine had an important side effect—its tendency to produce in some patients the facial and motor disturbances that are seen in Parkinson's disease. Modifications of chlorpromazine were developed in an effort to preserve the therapeutic benefit while avoiding this side effect, but—with very few exceptions—whenever an effective agent appeared it was also found to have the side effect. In addition to the phenothiazines, of which chlorpromazine was a member, an entirely new chemical class of drugs appeared, the butyrophenones, which were also effective in the treatment of schizophrenia but similarly suffered from the tendency to produce symptoms of Parkinsonism. An explanation of this phenomenon, however, had to await a better understanding of Parkinson's disease. This was not long in coming.

In 1960, a new technique was developed in Sweden for demonstrating certain neurotransmitters within the brain by means of their characteristic fluorescence under appropriate conditions. That technique was quickly applied by neuroanatomists and used within the brain to trace circuits that utilized these transmitters. A pathway that used dopamine as its transmitter was discovered in a region of the brain where lesions were known to exist in cases of Parkinsonism. This led to the hypothesis, and the ultimate demonstration, that in Parkinson's disease there is a partial destruction of the dopamine-containing nerve cells. Efforts to replenish the lost dopamine by administration of its precursor, L-Dopa, led to marked improvement in the patients, and represents one of the major contributions of fundamental neurological research to mental illness in recent times.

It was first suggested by Arvid Carlsson that antipsychotic drugs must block the effects of dopamine in the brain, which would explain their tendency to produce the symptoms of Parkinson's disease. On the basis of his studies and more recent observations on dopamine synapses in the brain and components of such synapses studied in vitro, it is now clear that Carlsson's insight was correct and that a major action of both the phenothiazine and the butyrophenone drugs is to diminish the actions of dopamine within the brain.

There is another drug that affects dopamine synapses —amphetamine—except that amphetamine exaggerates the effects of dopamine rather than diminishes them. Amphetamine is not at all an antipsychotic drug—quite the opposite. In animals it produces some of the behavior seen in schizophrenia—i.e., stereotyped movements of various kinds and aimless pacing. When it is abused

223

by human subjects, it produces a psychosis often indistinguishable from schizophrenia. The same drugs that are effective in the treatment of schizophrenia are also practically specific in terminating amphetamine psychosis, and amphetamine is known to exacerbate the psychosis of schizophrenic individuals. Thus, drugs that enhance dopamine activity in the brain tend to produce or aggravate schizophrenic symptoms, and those that diminish excessive dopamine activity are capable of relieving these symptoms. That does not mean that the biochemical disturbances underlying schizophrenia have been found in an abnormal overactivity of dopamine synapses. A therapeutic benefit may sometimes be obtained by an action that only indirectly affects the pathological process. It is nevertheless clear that continued and expanded research on the neurotransmitters in the brain cannot help contributing to our understanding of these illnesses. And with understanding will come more specific treatment and prevention.

What evidence do we have that a continued search for the biochemical factors of mental illness will be rewarding, or that such biochemical disturbances even exist? If there were clear evidence that these illnesses had important genetic bases, that would justify the search for their biochemical principles, because genetic factors must express themselves through biochemical processes.

Until quite recently, the evidence for the operation of genetic factors in these major mental illnesses was compelling but not conclusive, because nongenetic factors could account for the observation. Psychiatrists have known for a long time, and every epidemiological study has confirmed their observation, that the major mental illnesses run in families. There is an estimated 10-percent risk for the occurrence of schizophrenia in the parents, siblings, and offspring of schizophrenic individuals, and manic-depressive illness shows a comparable familial tendency. Although this figure is compatible with genetic transmission of these illnesses, it is not conclusive proof. Wealth and poverty run in families but are not genetically transmitted, and the familial occurrence of pellagra was used to support an erroneous genetic concept of what we now know to be essentially a nutritional disorder. A family shares not only its genetic endowments but also its environmental influences, and either or both of these factors may be responsible for familial disorders. Somewhat better evidence came from twin studies; a number of these studies have shown that for both schizophrenia and the affective disorders, a high risk (on the order of 50 percent) exists that the illness will appear in the identical twin of an affected person, while the risk for a fraternal twin is of the same order as that for a sibling. Because identical twins are derived from a single fertilized egg and are therefore the same genetically, whereas fraternal twins are no more than siblings conceived at the same time, the high concordance rates for these illnesses in identical twins would be expected in strongly genetic disorders, although that evidence is insufficient, in itself, to establish their genetic nature. Identical twins who look remarkably alike tend to be treated alike by their families and friends. They also share much of their environment and develop a mutual identification. It is probably factors such as these, rather than their genetic similarity, that account for the frequency with which identical twins choose the same occupation or marry similar partners.

During the past ten years a new approach has been used that appears to have succeeded in separating genetic from environmental factors in the transmission of schizophrenia. This approach consists of the study of adopted individuals who share their genetic endowment with their biological relatives, but their environment with their adoptive relatives. In the several studies that have been completed to date the results are quite consistent. Schizophrenia continues to run in families, but now its high prevalence is restricted to the genetic relatives of schizophrenics with whom they have shared few, if any, environmental factors. The adoptive relatives of schizophrenics who reared them and shared their environment show no more tendency to schizophrenia than does the population at large.

Recently evidence that some forms of manic and depressive illness have a genetic basis has been reported; in some families, these disorders have occurred in association with traits that reside in the X chromosome, such as color blindness and a specific blood group. Although this association does not occur in *all* families with manic-depressive illness, when it does occur, it follows a pattern so consistent that it would be difficult to explain on a nongenetic basis. One is forced to the conclusion that in the majority of severe cases of schizophrenia and in a substantial number of manic-depressive illnesses, genetic factors play a crucial causative role.

There thus exists the basis for a continued and intensified search for the biochemical processes through which these genetic factors operate in the development of the two most important forms of mental illness that confront us. In addition, neurobiology and psychobiology have in recent years provided important clues as to where to look, and powerful techniques have been developed and applied to this search. During this time a cohort of neurobiologists and psychiatrists has been trained, skilled in fundamental research and in clinical investigation. The time has never been more propitious or progress more promising for an understanding of these serious disturbances of the human mind.

The New
Orthomolecular Therapy
by Joann Rodgers

A seventy-three-year-old cancer patient becomes so irrational that he is consigned to a psychiatric ward after doctors decide that his malignancy has spread to the brain. After only four days on a regimen of vitamins B3 and C, he is discharged as "nearly normal."

A thirty-month-old Baltimore boy bites, screams himself hoarse daily, sleeps fewer than three hours a night, and tears up his mattress. It takes two aides to restrain him during a checkup. Diagnosed as a "brain allergy" victim, he is placed on a diet free of white sugar, white flour, cheese, and milk, and is given supplements of vitamins C, E, and B complex. Within six months, he sleeps through the night and is as self-controlled as any other three-year-old.

Mark Vonnegut, twenty-one, son of novelist Kurt Vonnegut, Jr., is a former schizophrenic who was once committed to a restraint ward. This fall, after a course of treatment based on vitamins B3, B6, B12, C, and E, and on folic acid, zinc sulphate, manganese, aspirin, antacids,

Joann Rodgers is a prizewinning medical writer and a syndicated medical columnist for the Hearst newspapers.

and lithium, young Vonnegut entered Harvard Medical School.

These patients are only a few of the thousands of American men, women, and children who depend on vitamins, minerals, nutrients such as wheat germ, and special diets for the cure of mental and emotional disorders ranging from psychosis to menstrual "blues." Similar treatments are advocated by some 800 "orthomolecular" psychiatrists and physicians, by hundreds of food faddists, "nutritional therapists," vitamin salesmen, and by a Nobel chemist. The regimens are available in a growing number of private clinics, federal, state, and municipal hospitals, private schools, doctors' offices, health-food stores, and pharmacies.

Schizophrenics, who fill more hospital beds than do all other mental patients combined, were the first on whom the new therapies were tried. Today, twenty years later, many practitioners prescribe megadoses of vitamins, low-sugar diets, electroshock therapy, and tranquilizers for a wide variety of other patients, including alcoholics, neurotics, depressives, the senile, and autistic and brain-damaged children.

These healers, who constitute a sort of psychiatric counterculture, insist that most abnormal behavior has no psychological "meaning." Such behavior, they say, is what happens when the brain is bathed in the wrong nutrients; thus aberrant behavior is a kind of cerebral pollution that can be cleared and corrected with the nutritionally "right" molecules (*ortho* is Greek for "right" and is the root of *orthomolecular*). Although psychological counseling is sometimes advocated, the aim of such treatment is to overcome bizarre "learned" behavior resulting from years of nutritional deficit and biochemical sabotage of the brain.

Nutritional therapists, whether physicians or laymen, embrace the medical model of mental illness. They cite genetic variation as the reason why not *all* nutritional

defectives are mentally ill. They promote their unortho-
dox theories and treatments in magazines, such as J. J.
Rodale's *Prevention;* scientific journals (unreferenced in
Index Medicus); popular books, such as Adelle Davis's *Eat
Right to Keep Fit,* Cheraskin and Ringsdorf's *Psychodietetics,*
and George Watson's *Nutrition and Your Mind.* The basic
textbook and treatise of the movement is *Orthomolecular
Psychiatry: Treatment of Schizophrenia,* which is the work of
Nobelist Linus Pauling and Dr. David Hawkins, director
of the North Nassau Mental Health Center in Manhasset,
New York, and President of the Academy of Ortho-
molecular Psychiatry.

According to the orthomolecular enthusiasts, the nation's overcrowded mental hospitals are monuments to
the failure of orthodox psychiatry

The American Psychiatric Association, the American
Medical Association, and half a dozen scientific panels
dismiss orthomolecular theories and practices as quack-
ery at worst and as unproved, experimental, "cookbook"
medicine at best.

An APA task force, headed by Dr. Morris Lipton, professor of psychiatry at the University of North Carolina,
concluded in 1973 that none of the claims made by orthomolecularists for the treatment of schizophrenia
could be confirmed by controlled clinical trials or repro-
duced by orthodox psychiatrists. It also scoffed at the
credit given vitamins in a treatment program that includes shock therapy and other tools of conventional
psychiatric care.

Dr. Thomas Ban, director of psychopharmacology at
McGill University and a member of the Lipton task force,
is now completing a twelve-part study of megavitamin
therapy among 350 schizophrenics in five hospitals. The
study is known in the field as the "goulash" trial, because
it incorporates a variety of orthomolecular prescriptions.
Ban's analysis is still under way at this writing. "I'll keep
an open mind until we have all the data in," says Ban.

229

"But it's true that earlier parts of the study found patients were not benefited by B3 or C (the bedrock of antischizophrenia therapy) and that some actually got worse."

Dr. Carl Pfeiffer, director of New Jersey's Brain Bio Center, a busy orthomolecular clinic, is young Vonnegut's doctor. He insists that orthomolecular and nutritional therapies benefit 90 percent of all his patients: "If [the task force] would do a fair trial, they'd get the same results we do."

Counterattacking, the orthodox medical establishment points out that orthomolecular specialists have been criminally prosecuted for fraud, censured by medical societies, and linked to patient deaths. One prominent therapist failed his psychiatric boards, and a University of California scientist found seventeen errors in a single speech by the late Adelle Davis. The orthomolecularists insist that the medical community just will not listen, so they must get the message to the public by any messengers they can recruit, even slightly tainted ones. Furthermore, nutritionists argue that "controlled trials" are beside the point. Patients, says Hawkins, "ain't mice or rats," and though he admits that no one knows why vitamin therapies work, "we have clinical proof that they do, and the public is making the decision in their favor."

Orthomolecular practitioners do, in fact, work from a clinical legacy in which diet produces spectacular effects on emotional and mental illness.

- Item: Some inherited metabolic disorders characterized by mental retardation, such as phenylketonuria, can be controlled with special diets.
- Item: In Greece, hospitalized schizophrenics improved when bread, which was a staple of their diets, became scarce under the Nazi occupation during World War II.
- Item: Vitamin-deficiency diseases, such as beriberi,

rickets, scurvy, and anemia, are often accompanied by chronic psychological disturbances, which disappear after nutritional therapy.

• Item: Menus rich in niacin (vitamin B3) sent thousands of institutionalized psychotics in the South home thirty years ago after their "mental" problems were traced to pellagra—a deficiency disease that was rampant among poor blacks who lived on diets heavy in corn meal and molasses.

In the early fifties, two Canadians, Drs. Abram Hoffer and J. Humphrey Osmond, suggested that "true" schizophrenia might be a deficiency disease as well, speculating, from various observations that schizophrenics may have a faulty metabolism that turns natural adrenalin into adrenochrome in the brain. Recalling the pellagra story and drawing on a vast knowledge of vitamin chemistry, the team administered massive amounts of B3 to schizophrenics so that the adrenochrome believed to be the cause of the disorder would be overcome and "neutralized." The first eight patients, the team reports, stayed well for fifteen years. Some 2,500 patients later, the Canadians claim a 90 percent "well" rate (an unverified statistic) and say incorporation of their treatment into conventional psychiatric care of the schizophrenic is the very least that "Establishment" medicine could do.

The Hoffer-Osmond regimen of niacin, vitamin C, pyridoxine, low-sugar diets, and tranquilizers has been given to thousands of patients, and disciples say that rehospitalization rates and suicide attempts have declined among these groups. The doctors also developed a biochemical test for "mauve" factor, a pink spot in the urine detectable by paper chromatography (a sort of sophisticated litmus-paper test).

Unfortunately for their own credibility, the adrenochrome that Osmond and Hoffer say is the cause of schizophrenia has never been isolated in a human, and

231

the "mauve" factor that they claim indicates schizophrenia has been found in many nonschizophrenics. Moreover, many psychological disorders have no consistent physiological markers that provide a parallel rationale for the Hoffer-Osmond theory.

Nevertheless, the orthomolecular and nutritional therapists continue their work undaunted. Pfeiffer, in his book *Mental and Elemental Nutrients,* reports that schizophrenia is, in fact, at least three distinct biochemical disorders that can be differentiated in blood and urine tests and on electroencephalogram tracings. And each of the three ailments requires different treatment:

Fifty percent of the "schizos" are, he says, paranoid schizophrenics with low levels of histamine, a compound released in the blood during allergic reactions. Twenty percent have *high* levels of histamine; these are the compulsive psychotics who are the "wrist cutters and overdosers." The remainder are those with "mauve" factor and/or "cerebral allergies."

At the Brain Bio Center, Pfeiffer treats the high-histamine group with vitamins, antihistamines, and psychotropic drugs. Those low in histamines also get vitamins and drugs as well as a high-protein diet. The mauve-factor group gets B6, zinc, lithium, vitamin E, and tranquilizers.

"I've chased . . . [schizophrenia] all my life, and we are finally fitting the pieces together," says Pfeiffer. His clinic now treats 1,500 patients, its operation dependent on endowments from grateful patients.

Orthodox neurochemistry holds that the brain removes oxygen, glucose, and amino acids, the basic building blocks of protein, from the bloodstream at a rate independent of alimentary activity, except in extreme starvation. Nutritional therapists dispute this concept and blame specific mental disorders on specific food deficits: paranoia, on low B12 absorption, for example; neurosis, on faulty sodium and potassium metabolism;

and alcoholism, anxiety, and aggressiveness, on abnormal sugar metabolism.

It is not difficult to dispute therapies promoted by faddists like Adelle Davis, who prescribes turnip greens and soybeans for nervous tension and Epsom salts, spinach and sea snails for "severe mental illness." Megavitamin and diet therapy is also vulnerable to criticism in terms of cost (initial workups can run to $500; pills, hundreds of dollars a year more) and safety (orthomolecular regimens have aggravated ulcers and have caused panic states and even death from overdoses and extreme dietary restrictions). Patients may also delay proved medical treatment because of the mistrust of all conventional therapy fostered by the orthomolecular movement. "We are dealing essentially with fanatics, and food is their religion," says Dr. Bernard T. Kaufman, chief of the National Institute of Health, Vitamin Metabolism Section.

The orthomolecular-nutritional position has survived such attacks and has been greatly strengthened by support of "defectors" from the ranks of orthodox medicine. Among them are Dr. Pfeiffer; Dr. Hoffer; Dr. Marshall Mandell, director of the New England Foundation for Allergic and Environmental Disease; Dr. Bernard Rimland, psychologist and senior navy scientist; Dr. Hawkins (Pauling's collaborator); and, finally, there is Pauling himself, who has done more than anyone else to legitimize megavitamin therapy.

Pauling, who is honorary president of the Academy of Orthomolecular Psychiatry, and who coined the term "orthomolecular psychiatry" almost twenty years ago, believes that brain tissue is so sensitive to changes in the molecular environment that mental problems result from nutritional insufficiencies long before any physical symptoms of nutritional deficiency occur. This "cerebral scurvy" or "pellagra" can be prevented, he claims, and cured, by "optimum concentrations of substances like vitamins C and B3 normally found in the body." Although Pauling's brilliance as a chemist gives him no credibility as a clinician or as a psychiatrist, his stature in the scientific community has lent considerable authority to the many recent research and therapeutic claims of the nutritional specialists. These claims and therapies include:

- The use of zinc and manganese for the control of senile dementia, a condition they say can be diagnosed from low blood levels of spermine, a naturally occurring nerve stimulant.
- The removal of certain foods (grasses, dairy products, sugar, caffeine, yeast, citrus, and artificial flavorings and colorings containing salicylates) for the control of hyperactivity, depression, fatigue, paranoia, and phobias among victims of cerebral allergies. (These views are developed at length by Dr. Carlton Fredericks in his book *Psychonutrition.*)
- Turning hyperactive behavior on and off like a light switch in some children by surreptitiously removing salicylates from their favorite diet of cereals, hot dogs, ice cream, soft drinks, and chocolate. Dr. Ben Feingold, a San Francisco allergist, uses this technique to prove the case for cerebral allergy.
- Dietary control of functional hypoglycemia, a chronic low-blood-sugar condition, for the cure of schizophrenia, alcoholism, and antisocial behavior. The AMA calls hypoglycemia a rare disorder; orthomolecularists say it afflicts 10 percent of the population. Some hypoglycemics do display emotional problems. "So do some people with big feet," carps one critic.
- The use of vitamins and antihypoglycemic diets for the cure of a craving for alcohol. Dr. Hawkins claims the majority of 600 alcoholics he has treated since 1966 have done well on this regimen. Dr. Rimland

claims dramatic improvement for autistic or aggressive children on megavitamins as well.

• The psychiatric establishment complains that all the anecdotal "case history" evidence in the world still doesn't add up to a grain of scientific evidence in support of nutritional therapy for mental illness.

• "I have seen really sick patients get better on injections of sterile water," says Dr. Robert Gibson, president-elect of the APA and director of the prestigious Sheppard-Pratt hospital. "One can't underestimate the placebo effect of caring, inherent in all forms of therapy, that could well explain the benefits these people claim for their patients."

It may not be that simple, however. Some principles of orthomolecular theory are reasonable, and bits and pieces are being validated by orthodox researchers. Dr. Seymour Kety of Harvard and Dr. William Bunney of the National Institute of Mental Health believe that there is now conclusive evidence of a genetic influence in schizophrenia. Genes are linked to enzymes, and the conclusion these doctors have reached supports a biochemical basis for some forms of mental illness.

Experiments have also shown that the transmission of nerve impulses in the brain may be chemically triggered, rather than electrically sparked as current scientific texts maintain.

Dr. John Freeman and his team at Johns Hopkins University, for example, have successfully treated a fifteen-year-old schizophrenic catatonic girl born with homocystinuria, a metabolic defect. Biochemical tests disclosed a vitamin deficiency linked to another disorder known to respond to treatment with folic acid and vitamin B6. Therapy with these nutrients cleared her of psychotic symptoms, including hallucinations. Although the metabolic disorder did not alone cause her psychosis (her sister has homocystinuria too, but no mental illness) the possibility that brain chemistry plays a significant role in common mental disorders is bolstered by such work.

Says Dr. Richard Jed Wyatt, acting head of the National Institute of Mental Health, "The concepts of orthomolecular psychiatry are attractive and stimulating." And some recent research findings are consistent with their concepts.

Unfortunately, evidence to support orthomolecular theories *is* still weak, and the unorthodox methods used make it difficult to verify the claims made by their advocates in any way that would satisfy the medical establishment; so any "final" pronouncements must await future developments.

Medicine
for Melancholy
— • —
by Anthony Wolff

Some people are depressed most of the time; most people are depressed some of the time: all told, depression is the most common emotional illness of mankind. An expert of the National Institute of Mental Health recently testified that between 5 and 10 million people in the United States alone are "seriously" depressed, while millions more suffer milder symptoms without ever being counted. The NIMH estimates that 20 million Americans—10 percent of the population—experience a "clinically depressed" mood every year. Clearly, the discovery and development in recent years of several families of chemicals that can ease depression's symptoms raises the hope of relief for tens of millions of previously hopeless sufferers. Ironically, however, the promise of a chemical cure for depression, enthusiastically promoted by some specialists and their grateful patients, has reopened some fundamental and long-standing questions about what depression is and what to do about it. The resulting public controversy

Anthony Wolff is a free-lance writer who contributes regularly to *Saturday Review* and other magazines.

and confusion has damped the general applause for a new medical miracle.

While their depressive patients suffered, doctors have been debating the causes and cures of the ailment since long before Hippocrates himself wrote the first clinical description of "melancholia" almost 2,500 years ago. Yet, for a disease that has been so popular for so long, depression remains stubbornly mysterious. Even today, the best experts don't know what causes it; they don't agree on the proper classification of its many manifestations; they are not even sure that there is a single disease behind depression's disparate symptoms. It is no wonder, then, that the public is even more confused than its physicians and that there are questions about chemicals that treat the symptoms of depression while ignoring the nature of the disease and its causes.

Much of the confusion can be ascribed to the peculiar personality of the disease itself. The depressive's complaints can be deceptively diverse and ambiguously common. They range all the way from a general sadness and lack of *joie de vivre,* to loss of appetite, inability to concentrate or make decisions, insomnia and waning sexual interest, all the way to suicidal despair. Moreover, while the depressive's suffering is unimpeachably real and excruciating, his primary symptoms are all subjective. Depression is "all in the mind"—as the victim's friends and loved ones are wont to reassure him, trying to be helpful but only making the pain worse—and there is nothing to be seen, measured, excised, or exorcised.

Throughout human history, one of the typical depressive's most devastating conceits has been the unshakable conviction that there is no end to his agony, no relief for his suffering, no help for him. (Or for her, more probably. For reasons that are unknown, and thus susceptible to endless ideological argument, depression seems to occur in women much more frequently than it does in men.) Until the advent of the antidepressant chemicals, even the relatively few depressives who found professional help risked having their worst fears confirmed. Ever since Freud, the orthodox treatment for depression —indeed, the only real treatment—has been a long course of psychoanalysis or some derivative therapy in search of an unresolved emotional conflict presumed to be the ultimate cause of the trouble. But even for the fortunate few with the necessary time and money and access to a talented analyst or therapist, the prognosis has been uncertain at best.

Now, with the new chemicals, claims one of their most prominent exponents, Dr. Ronald R. Fieve of New York's Columbia-Presbyterian Medical Center, depression has become "a relatively easy and gratifying disorder to treat." The antidepressant drugs have inspired a new psychiatric subspecialty, called psychopharmacology, which boasts that for the first time in medical history there are specific medicines that are effective against an emotional illness in as many as 80 percent of cases. Any further recourse to traditional psychoanalysis and the other "talking therapies" in cases of depression, insist the more militant psychopharmacologists, is even more than before a waste of time and money. Depression expert Dr. Nathan S. Kline, director of research at New York's Rockland State Hospital, recently told a TV talk-show audience that from now on not only depression but "the great majority of emotional diseases can be treated chemically." Only patients with "milder" problems, people whose "coping mechanisms aren't functioning," will have any need of traditional psychotherapy, and then only after their depression has been chemically cured. "Traditional psychotherapy and analysis," agrees Dr. Fieve, "will become, for the most part, obsolete." The analyst's fifty-minute hours, he predicted in a recent interview, will be reserved for those who "don't have anyone else to talk to" about relatively minor and superficial complaints.

Where traditional psychiatry has erred for so long, according to Kline and Fieve, is in assuming that depression's emotional symptoms must have an emotional cause. "I have no quarrel with psychotherapy," insists Kline, but "in most cases of clinical depression, I believe it is fundamentally a biochemical disorder." Depression, says Kline, is "a biochemical accident" that "in most cases is very probably triggered by some disarray in the biochemical tides that sweep back and forth within the body." In most cases, echoes Fieve, "the origin of the moodswing"—his term for a whole catalog of emotional changes—"is physical, metabolic, and chemical." The sufferer can be reassured that "it is not the problems in his past that are causing the moodswing." Depression is a chemical problem, conclude the doctors; it demands a chemical response.

In shifting not only the treatment of a major mental illness but also its very definition from the emotional to the physical—from the invisible "mind" to the corporeal brain—the psychopharmacologists maintain that they are only filling a prescription written by Freud himself. Even as he was advancing his psychoanalytic interpretation of mental illness, Freud realized that "the shortcomings of our descriptions would probably disappear if for the psychological ones we could . . . substitute physiological or chemical ones." In practice, he predicted, "the future may teach us how to exercise a direct influence by means of particular chemical substances."

Still early in the "future" that Freud foresaw, the psychopharmacologists have three families of drugs that combine marked antidepressant effects and manageable or tolerable side effects. Two groups, the monoamine oxidase (MAO) inhibitors and the tricyclics, are effective in cases of simple, "unipolar" depression; while lithium carbonate, the third, is uniquely and dramatically potent in blocking the manic phase of "bipolar" depression, a bizarre form in which uncontrollable emotional "highs"

240

alternate with the typical "lows." The usual course of treatment begins with the doctor trying various drugs and dosages to find the appropriate combination. Then, several weeks may pass while the chemicals build up to an effective level in the brain. Once the chemical takes hold, maximum relief may take another month or two, after which patients subject to recurring attacks are reduced to a lower, maintenance dosage.

As is so often the case in medicine, the pragmatic clinical use of the antidepressant drugs is running far ahead of the research that will one day explain why and how they work and allow them to be used with more predictable effectiveness and accuracy. Meanwhile, however, some of the psychopharmacologists, with Kline and Fieve in the vanguard, have become impatient at what they consider the unreasonable reluctance of many of their colleagues to enlist in what Fieve describes as a "revolution in psychiatry." "The general public, as well as most physicians and many psychiatrists," Fieve complains, "still do not understand what depression is—how to diagnose it and how to apply satisfactory drug treatment." According to Kline, "depression is both the most frequent and the most undertreated of all psychiatric disorders."

Part of the problem, as Fieve sees it, is that most doctors don't recognize depressions when they see them. Diagnosis is complicated by depression's talent for masquerading in a confusing variety of symptoms, both physical and emotional, perfectly mimicking everything from alcoholism to lower-back pains. "Patients come in complaining of various types of aches and pains," a general practitioner in the Tennessee mountains recently reported, "but when you get into it, you don't find any real physical reason for it. Frequently when you treat the patient with an antidepressant drug, it will relieve their pains."

Even among psychiatrists, Fieve charges, the frequency of incorrect diagnosis is "shocking." He cites a study of nine New York–area hospitals in which "86 percent of depressions and manic depressions were, in fact, given other labels"—most often schizophrenia—and mistreated accordingly.

Dr. Fieve is even more critical of his colleagues' failure to prescribe drug therapy when they do recognize depression. The idea that drugs can relieve depression quickly and cheaply, he charges, is "a threat to psychiatry's traditional and costly ways of treating mood disorders." In the case of lithium therapy, in which he has played a leading role as researcher and advocate for more than fifteen years, Fieve suggests, "One might even postulate that the world economic market for treating moodswing was now being threatened by a simple and inexpensive salt that could not be marketed with any great profit to anyone." Many of his colleagues, Fieve stated in a recent interview, have a vested interest in careers and self-esteem founded on outmoded approaches to depression, and they resist change. "There's a lag time of twenty years," he complained, "in getting our research into Park Avenue psychiatrists' offices."

In an effort to short-cut what they regard as the slow, circuitous path of progress, both Fieve and Kline have decided—quite independently—to take their cases directly to the public. They have become the stars of a mass-media medicine show, sitting for interviews and giving headline-yielding speeches, writing popular books and magazine manifestos, and appearing on television talk shows, in an apparent campaign to turn the issue of depression therapy into a popular referendum.

Amplified by an attentive and respectful press, the doctors have been getting their message across to millions who didn't know a unipolar depression from a unicycle before. Presumably, they have been making converts to the cause of chemical therapy. Among their colleagues, however, the doctors' public performances

have drawn some negative, even angry, reviews and pro-
voked a storm of protest in the professional press. Professional etiquette prohibits doctors from criticizing one
another in public. In private, however, and often not for
attribution, many well-qualified psychiatrists charge that
Fieve and Kline are overselling their chemicals to a public that is eager for easy answers to difficult questions.
The critics include psychoanalysts with long experience
in treating depression, as well as psychiatrists who eclec-
tically employ antidepressant chemicals in some cases
but not in others.

"It's not true that depression comes from nothing,"
insists Dr. Silvano Arieti, a psychoanalyst and professor
at New York Medical College, who edited the mul-
tivolume *American Handbook of Psychiatry* and won the National Book Award for his *Interpretation of Schizophrenia.*
"There is *always* a psychological reason for depression."
Treating a psychological pain with drugs, says Arieti, is
"like taking a drug for a toothache instead of going to the
dentist. Drug therapy is purely symptomatic. Psychotherapy is indispensable for complete recovery."

The very title of Dr. Fieve's book, *Moodswing,* and his
use of that both simple and suggestive term to cover all
degrees of manic depression, has been criticized as an
invitation to normal readers to imagine that the book is
describing them. The reader's impression may be
strengthened when Fieve asserts that "chemically treatable mood disorders can now be easily recognized in
normal people"; or later, when Fieve asks rhetorically,
"What about the millions of people who just seem to be
getting on in life, with day-to-day, humdrum existences
in which they don't seem to have any energy for anything
—the apathetic, the bored, those who don't seem to be
getting any pleasure out of living?" Readers who recognize themselves in that hazy mirror may well be suffering,
says Fieve, "from mild forms of chemically treatable depression."

Dr. Fieve's special interest, however, is not in the simple depressions of ordinary people. His preoccupation—and the subject of his pioneering research—is manic depression and, especially, its control with lithium. Much of *Moodswing* is devoted to making a case for an intimate connection between manic depression and creative energy in the arts, politics, and business. Abraham Lincoln, Winston Churchill, Ralph Nader, and ITT president Harold Geneen: superachievers all, and all manic-depressives, according to Fieve. A touch of mania can boost such talents to spectacular heights, Fieve claims. When the "high" gets too high or the depressive phase takes over, however, a little lithium is what the doctor orders.

There is no longer any significant argument about the use of lithium against the manic phase of manic depression. It is dramatically effective, and it has been approved by the Food and Drug Administration for that use—but for that use only. Fieve maintains, however, and Kline agrees, that lithium is also effective in controlling recurrent unipolar, or simple, depression. Psychiatrists who disagree, Fieve says, "haven't worked with lithium" or haven't kept up with the latest research.

But the control of depression, simple and manic, Fieve suggests in his book, may be only the beginning of lithium's talents. The common mineral salt, he hints, has shown early promise of effectiveness against alcoholism, adolescent behavior disorders, cancer, and menstrual depression, among other assorted ills. "As yet," Fieve teases, "we do not know if lithium is essential for normal biological processes"; and he takes the prudent position that "lithium should not, on the basis of the present evidence, be added to the water supplies," but only after he has considered "the fascinating possibility."

Fieve's enthusiasm—even passion—for lithium scares a lot of doctors who readily endorse the use of antidepressant chemicals, including lithium, when they are indicated, but who find little comfort in the prospect of lithium in major quantities in the hands of a broad public. The problem is not that lithium is an addictive or intoxicating substance; it isn't. But, unlike the other antidepressants, lithium is extremely toxic. Moreover, the therapeutic and toxic levels are so close that the concentration of lithium in the blood must be monitored at least monthly during the entire course of therapy. The patient must be constantly on the alert for a variety of side effects —tremors, nausea, blurred vision or speech, diarrhea, and others—that might signal lithium poisoning. An acute toxic reaction can end in coma and death if emergency treatment is not administered promptly. Lithium is especially dangerous for patients with cardiovascular or kidney disease, or for those on salt-free diets or diuretics.

In sum, a lot of responsible, respected psychotherapists think Kline and Fieve are going too far too fast in their public campaign to encourage doctors to diagnose depression more frequently and to administer antidepressant drugs more readily. At the same time, there are tens of thousands of depression-prone patients who can testify that the antidepressant drugs have banished their black, waking nightmares and restored them to functioning, productive lives.

Can Psychiatry
Save the Republic?

by Arthur Schlesinger, Jr.

Among other perennial burdens, the plain people of the
world have long had to suffer the possibility that those
who rule over them might turn out to be lunatics. From
the Neros, Caligulas, and Heliogabaluses of the Roman
Empire to the Hitlers and Stalins, the Duvaliers and
Amins, of our own enlightened age, deranged men have
wielded the power of the state—men whose relations to
reality were at best intermittent and whose energies, at
least in the view of their victims, might have found better
outlets by weaving baskets at the funny farm. For most
of history this possibility of living under the rod of a
madman was one more uncontrollable statistical risk,
like the hazard of hurricanes or of the plague. In recent
times the risk has come to seem unendurable—partly
because the rise of democracy has instilled the idea that
rulers are accountable to the ruled; partly because the
rise of psychiatry has created the impression that madness is readily identifiable and occasionally curable;
mostly, perhaps, because the risk of madness at the pin-
nacle is no longer minor when science and technology

Dr. Arthur Schlesinger, Jr., is Albert Schweitzer Professor of Humanities at
the City University of New York and the author of *The Imperial Presidency*.

have handed rulers the power to blow up the planet.

We are all disconcerted, to put it mildly, by the awareness of the defenselessness of our civilization before the unconscious wishes, drives, and obsessions of persons possessing vast power. Nor can Americans comfortably regard this any longer as a problem peculiar to dictatorships across the seas. As our own political order has increasingly concentrated in the Presidency, and as recent Presidents have broken out of the constitutional system of accountability, we Americans live more than ever at the mercy of presidential caprice and compulsion. Once this process got under way, whether out of disagreeable coincidence or masochistic gratification, we elected in quick succession (1964, 1968) the two most capricious and compulsive Presidents we have ever had.

Is there nothing we can do about this vulnerability to the psychological vagaries of our rulers? For, despite the resignation of Richard Nixon, our lives are going to continue to rest in the hands of individuals who command the state. It is true that institutions have purposes of their own and often succeed in dominating those presumed to run them. But let no one suppose that institutions themselves cannot be dominated when the man on top is sufficiently able or determined (that is, compulsive without being manifestly certifiable). Adolf Hitler forced the mighty *Reichswehr* into a course of defeat and disaster. We cannot count on institutions to serve us.

The American government, of course, is no dictatorship. Still, Clark Clifford has accurately described the executive branch as a chameleon, taking its color and values from the personality of the President. Moreover, the very extent of presidential power, the myth and majesty of the office, the easy isolation it brings, the sedulous sycophancy that surrounds it—all intensify the strain on such normality and stability as rulers may initially take into the White House. Because all this is so,

247

the presidential personality, the pattern of the presidential unconscious, becomes a matter of public significance. And, with the emergence of psychiatry as an aggressive cultural force, the question has arisen whether psychiatrists cannot rescue us from the psychopathology of power—whether psychiatric insights and methods will not bring reliable control of the presidential psyche.

This inquiry necessarily raises a prior question: whether what Freud liked to call the "science of the unconscious" really offers solid basis for guidance, selection, and constraint in public affairs. The eminent public servant and historian Herbert Feis, invited to consider the claims of the psychoanalytical interpretation of history, defined the problem when he asked the tough questions: "How adequate psychological knowledge is, how stable it is, how precise it is, and how agreed it is." Freud himself in expansive moments said that the hypothesis of the unconscious "paves the way to a decisive new orientation in the world" and would become "indispensable to all the sciences which are concerned with the evolution of human civilization." But he was not describing the present state of the art; he was predicting its future. In the years since Freud's death, however, psychiatrists —or at least a highly vocal minority among them—have decided that the future is here and are demanding their inheritance. Their art, they insist, has progressed to the point where it must be summoned to a controlling place in public affairs. Nor is it easy to deny, after the recent American experience, the strong national interest in keeping out of government persons whose psychic agitations may withdraw them from reality and disable them from rational decision.

The psychiatric invasion of public affairs has sought to embrace both irrationalities sweeping through masses of people and neuroses afflicting individuals. "Psychohistory" and "psychobiography" carry psychiatric techniques back into the past; proposals for psychiatric control of collective or individual psychopathology project them into the future. As long ago as 1941 Dr. George H. Stevenson in his presidential address before the American Psychiatric Association indulged himself in the large hope that "when the history of our second century comes to be written, may it be recorded that the American Psychiatric Association was largely responsible for the elimination of the international psychosis, war." After the Second World War, Dr. Brock Chisholm, another eminent Canadian psychiatrist and the head of the World Health Organization, argued that war could be cured if only psychiatrists were empowered to teach mothers how to love their babies. The intentions of Drs. Stevenson and Chisholm—and of later psychiatrists who adopted their tone and expectation—were generous and admirable. The claims they made for psychiatry were perhaps immodest.

Little in the literature or in clinical experience encourages the idea that psychiatry can provide the means even to explain mass psychopathology, much less to control it. Psychiatric explanations in this field tend to be dangerously reductive, too often omitting from consideration the external sources of social disorientation and disorder. Many psychiatrists let loose in history or current affairs forget the point so clearly made by another American Psychiatric Association president, Dr. Raymond W. Waggoner. He reminded his colleagues of the distinction "between *realistic conflict,* characterized as it is by incompatibility of values and interests and by differing means and ends, and *nonrealistic conflict,* which is the product of tension release, projected hostility, historical traditions, and sheer ignorance and error." The abiding psychiatric fallacy is to suppose that politics consists essentially of imagined, rather than real, issues.

In recent years it has been on the second front—the psychic troubles of individual political leaders—that psychiatrists have been especially aggressive. The idea of long-distance psychoanalysis has come into vogue. There was that singularly foolish intervention of psychiatrists in the 1964 presidential election when 1,846 members of the American Psychiatric Association—11 percent of the whole—delivered solemn diagnoses of the mental state of Senator Barry Goldwater, a man who had rested on none of their couches and whom most of them had never seen. Perhaps because psychiatrists are immune to libel actions once their subjects are dead, they display even greater confidence in psychoanalyzing historical figures.

The New York Times op-ed page gave space not long ago to the sagacities of Dr. Russel V. Lee of the Stanford Medical School. Dr. Lee began in a jocose vein: "In a democratic regime the very qualities of egocentricity and megalomania, characteristic of many psychoses, are precisely those that lead men to aspire to high office. In fact, there are those who say that the very fact of aspiration to high office is *ipso facto* proof of mental derangement. I would not go so far." At least I trust Dr. Lee was being jocose, though the wit is of the same order as the counter gag that psychiatrists go into the profession because they are afraid of their own craziness. After his pleasantries, Dr. Lee got down to business, dismissing Napoleon as a "diminutive, strutting paranoiac," Lloyd George as "probably a manic-depressive," Woodrow Wilson as "not mentally sound," Orlando of Italy as "a nothing," Kaiser Wilhelm II as a "strutting, ridiculous, adult adolescent," and so on through history.

Why, a layman is bound to wonder, is Dr. Lee so hung up on the word *strutting?* There are those who might say —I would not go so far—that the good doctor comes on as a pretty mean strutter, too, airily disposing of historical figures, most of them rather more considerable persons than he is himself, and propounding a simpleminded explanation of problems that have bedeviled historians for years, such as the origins of the First World

War. Dr. Lee's conclusion is dismally predictable: "All public officials should be required to have . . . comprehensive psychological testing" once a year, with the tests presumably to be administered by professors at the Stanford Medical School. That no doubt would have saved the world from Wilson and Lloyd George.

Two recent proposals elaborate this principle of all power to the psychiatrists (or, depending on sectarian inflection, to the psychologists). I recognize that neither of the authors of these particular schemes, both of which have received considerable publicity, is a member of the American Psychiatric Association. Still, many members of that association endorse the basic principle of these plans—that the psychological expert should be empowered to sit in judgment over the democratic process.

One proposal comes from a distinguished psychologist and a most valued citizen of New York City, Dr. Kenneth Clark, in his presidential address to the American Psychological Association in 1971. Dr. Clark, whose secular activities I greatly admire, is not much concerned, it must be said, with the "science of the unconscious." He is, I judge, closer in spirit to Skinner than to Freud. But, however much Freudians and Skinnerites, psychoanalysts and behaviorists, dispute everything else, they unite in preferring the priesthood to the laity. Thus Dr. Clark begins by saying that the traditional modes by which power has been controlled—religion, moral philosophy, law, education—can no longer be relied upon to contain man's "primitive and egocentric behavior." The old modes left too wide a margin of error; in the nuclear age a single error could terminate the life of man on Earth. We must therefore hasten to develop "that degree of precision, predictability, and moral control essential to the survival of man." So far, I take it, many psychiatrists would agree with Dr. Clark. Most would disagree, I presume, with his remedy; for Dr. Clark's faith is that we may well be "on the threshold of that type

251

of scientific biochemical intervention which could stabilize and make dominant the moral and ethical propensities of man and subordinate, if not eliminate, his negative and primitive behavioral tendencies." He would therefore impose as a requirement upon all political leaders that "they accept and use the earliest perfected form of psychotechnological, biochemical intervention which would assure their positive use of power and reduce or block the possibility of their using power destructively." And so "psychotechnological medication" would usher humankind into a new era—though whether that era is more accurately forecast in *Walden Two* or in *A Clockwork Orange* one cannot at this point be sure.

Dr. Arnold A. Hutschnecker, I understand, is an internist by training. But in recent years he has infiltrated psychiatry, where he is now campaigning for what he calls "psychopolitics." Dr. Hutschnecker adorns his campaign with the usual psychohistorical nonsense. "What torture and misery could have been spared . . . the world," he writes, if Woodrow Wilson "could have had competent psychiatric help before slipping into the darkness of his depression." Or if Abraham Lincoln "could have been helped to understand the nature of the anguish produced by his inner conflicts . . . perhaps there would not have been any need for the bloody killings of the Civil War." Poor old Lincoln! Psychiatrists find such pleasure in citing his passages of melancholy in order to pronounce him a hopeless neurotic. One cannot doubt that Lincoln had his low periods. "A tendency to melancholy," he wrote as a young man, ". . . let it be observed, is a misfortune, not a fault." But I also note that Freud himself said, "I have to be somewhat miserable in order to write well."

The historian can only find breathtaking the certitude with which Drs. Lee and Hutschnecker announce their historical verdicts. They seem to find no objective problems in public affairs, only imagined problems. But—no

252

kidding, fellows—the Civil War was not fought because of Lincoln's neuroses. It was fought because of the determination of the Southern states to perpetuate an indefensible institution called slavery. No amount of psychiatric exorcism could have done away with intractable issues existing outside Lincoln's psyche in 1861, any more than the successful analysis of Wilson could have done away, say, with Imperial Germany's unrestricted submarine warfare.

Dr. Hutschnecker will have none of this. The problem of deranged rulers can be solved, he assures us, if two steps are taken. One is to empower a panel of psychiatrists, chosen by the profession, to administer the Hartman Value Profile to all contenders for the Presidency and award those who pass the test "mental health certificates . . . similar to the Wasserman test demanded by states before marriage." The second is to establish a resident psychiatrist in the White House to watch over the mental health of the President and his staff. Do not psychiatrists understand that their negative judgment of Lincoln, for example, is hardly an argument for assigning them the authority to screen future Presidents? Would it have been a triumph for the republic if Dr. Hutschnecker and his panel had been able to flunk Lincoln on the Hartman Value Profile and keep him out of the White House? If this is what psychiatry has to tell us about Lincoln, one can say only, as Lincoln said of Grant's addiction to whiskey, that some of our more recent Presidents should have had Lincoln's addiction to melancholy.

The most arresting aspect of such proposals is the light they throw on the psychiatrists who make them. As James Wechsler, whose moving book *In a Darkness* should be required reading for every psychiatrist, wisely commented, "What is perhaps most vulnerable about [Dr. Hutschnecker's] essay is the intimation that he or his counterparts might have so decisive a bearing on history." It may be, Dr. Lee, that egocentricity and megalo-mania are not the monopoly of politicians.

One wonders what Freud himself would have made of all this. Despite moments of programmatic euphoria, Freud was a careful man. He did not live long enough to see the rise of psychohistory; but, although he would not quite say that the attempt "to carry psychoanalysis over into the cultural community was absurd or doomed to be fruitless," he enjoined caution and implied skepticism. Those who try to psychoanalyze social groups, he said, must never forget that they are "only dealing with analo-gies and that it is dangerous, not only with men but also with concepts, to tear them from the sphere in which they have originated and been evolved."

Even in the analysis of individuals, Freud knew that his method had limits. One doubts whether he would have been much impressed by the call for psychiatric examina-tions of public officials. He understood, as one president of the American Psychiatric Association, Dr. Judd Mar-mor, has put it, that, while physical examinations require only the patient's passive presence, "an adequate psychi-atric examination requires his wholehearted cooopera-tion. . . . We know only too well from clinical experience that if a patient is determined to conceal or dissemble, an adequate psychiatric diagnosis can often be rendered impossible." Freud understood too that even with wholehearted cooperation, problems might exist beyond the reach of the method. The creative process perplexed him particularly. "The nature of artistic attainment," he said at one point, is ". . . psychoanalytically inaccessible to us." He summed it up in his essay on Dostoevski: "Before the problem of the creative artist, analysis must lay down its arms."

A significant admission. For of all historic figures, art-ists live most freely out of their unconscious. Their crea-tions are filled with clues for the analyst. Paintings and poems reveal more than state papers do. Freud's own

254

essays on artists are brilliantly suggestive. But men of power are harder nuts to crack. Freud himself proved this. His greatest disaster was his inquiry into politics when, with his former patient, William C. Bullitt, he wrote a biography of Wilson. If analysis must lay down its arms before the creative artist, what must it do before that far more shuttered and guarded figure, the practical politician?

And Freud was one of the incomparables. He was a man of subtle and penetrating intelligence, possessed by an epic poetic-scientific vision. That vision has decomposed since his death. Russel Lee, Arnold Hutschnecker, and Kenneth Clark all would like to clear our rulers, approving some, rejecting others. But they cannot agree among themselves on the criteria of diagnosis and prescription. Few professional communities are so riddled with dissension. Dr. Karl Menninger, one of the patriarchs, confessed a few years ago, "I give you the assurance that I don't understand a good deal of what my colleagues are talking about." Entire conventions of psychiatrists are given over to discussing the questions raised by Herbert Feis—the questions of the adequacy, stability, precision, and consensus of psychological knowledge. Yet these are the people who, while they argue so fiercely among themselves, exhort a distraught and consequently credulous public to give them veto power over the democratic process.

What has a historian, whose ambition is merely to record the actions of human beings, to say to those whose pretension is to search their souls? Only perhaps that the searching of souls is a tricky undertaking—and it may well be as tricky for the searchers as for the searched. Those whose calling requires them to believe that they have the key to the psyche of others must, one would think, be all the more resolute in their own discipline, in their own skepticism of self, in their own sense of limitation and humility. The life of affairs is not just the projection of delusions on a social screen. Public issues are not just figments in the imagination of politicians. Problems do exist. They are real. One must add that politics is fully as sophisticated a field of psychiatry, requiring quite as much specialized knowledge and trained instinct—even if politicians, unlike psychiatrists, do not dress up their black arts in a technical vocabulary.

No one can deny the necessity for finding methods by which people may be protected from the psychic agitations and obsessions of their rulers. But one doubts whether the program of all power to the psychiatrists is really the most reliable means by which to restore the American Presidency to reality. "Sometimes," Jefferson said in his first inaugural address, "it is said that man cannot be trusted with the government of himself. Can he, then, be trusted with the government of others? Or have we found angels in the forms of kings to govern him?" Replacing *kings* by *psychiatrists* does not dispose of Jefferson's question. The proposal of psychiatric clearance, so lightly demanded by the psychopoliticians, has extraordinary implications for the whole idea of democracy and self-government. The theory of the divine right of psychiatrists is quite as destructive as absolute monarchy itself of the right affirmed in the Declaration of Independence and the Constitution—the right of men and women to govern themselves by freely choosing their rulers.

There are other ways besides psychiatric testing to restore the Presidency to reality—ways that sustain democracy and that, indeed, have worked well enough for most of American history. What has constrained the presidential psyche during the life of the republic has been the political and institutional setting in which the President has operated. The Founding Fathers had two purposes. One was to create a strong and effective national government. The second was to keep that government within a strong and effective system of accountability. Accountability means, of course, scrutiny, challenge, criticism. It means these things not just once every four years but as a continuous part of the process of democracy, expressed not just through quadrennial elections but in the daily workings of government. Few Presidents have relished scrutiny, challenge, and criticism. In this respect they have been like historians; even perhaps like psychiatrists. But up to very recent times, nearly all have accepted the discipline of consent.

The constitutional system of accountability had one grave weakness: the realm of foreign affairs. In responding to presidential initiatives in foreign policy, Congress, the courts, and the people felt much less sure of their ground, much less confident of their information and judgment, and were therefore much less inclined to challenge and check and balance, as they did so freely in domestic affairs. The more active a role the United States took in the world, the less responsibility Congress wished to assume (especially after its disastrous record when it tried to run foreign affairs between the two world wars) and the more power flowed to Presidents, who characteristically accepted it as their due. As foreign policy tempted Presidents to break out of the system of accountability, the Presidency perhaps began to seem a refuge to personalities on whom accountability exacted an intolerable psychic toll. Johnson and Nixon ultimately gave the impression that they saw the process of scrutiny, challenge, and criticism not just as unfair—all Presidents tend to do that—but as illegitimate. They began to build a high wall around the office. The presidential unconscious, once contained by the historic modes of accountability, became more free than ever before to assert itself against the reality principle.

One doubts whether the way to reestablish the reality principle in the White House is to give the President a psychiatrist-in-residence as company behind the high wall. The thing to do rather is to level the wall. Who after all will choose the White House psychiatrist? The President would end up either with a Rasputin or a stooge. Or is the idea to make it a post subject to senatorial confirmation? The whole project crumbles under examination. Plainly the democratic way to induce Presidents to confront reality is simply to enforce the system of accountability. We can begin by abandoning the latter-day notion that election to the Presidency transforms a second-rate politician into a minor, or major, divinity. The theory of the transsubstantiation of the Presidency must be secularized. The singular idea embodied in Nixon's idiot phrase about "respect for the Presidency" —a phrase that no previous President, so far as I can discover, found it necessary to use—must be sent back to the monarchical societies from which it comes. ("History does not look kindly on regicide," said Hugh Scott, the Republican leader in the Senate, in warning his colleagues against impeaching Nixon. At what point, one wondered, had the President of the United States become a king?) All Presidents are entitled to full courtesy, as is every other citizen in the land. But no President is entitled to any more respect than his words and actions earn him. "There is no worse heresy," wrote Lord Acton, "than that the office sanctifies the holder of it."

Richard Nixon was hardly the first President whose case history excited the professional curiosity of psychiatrists. But earlier Presidents were limited in the extent to which they could work out their personal problems at the expense of the country—limited by the strength of a system of accountability that they could not ignore. They remained more or less tethered to the reality principle, not because they benefited from psychiatric attention but because they could not escape the obligations of explanation and persuasion. They had no choice but to take the views of others into account—the views of Congress, of the courts, of their colleagues in the executive branch, of their political party, of newspapers, of national opinion. They could not vault over the discipline of consent. All this kept them in touch with the real world. It was only the decay of the system of accountability under pressure of international crisis that made possible the rise of the solipsistic Presidency. And if we want to restore the Presidency to reality, we must begin by encouraging future Presidents to respect the system of accountability. The way to do this was thoughtfully provided by the Founding Fathers.

For the men who gathered in Philadelphia 190 years ago were not fools or innocents. They had a hard understanding of human nature. They understood power—both that it was essential and that it was liable to abuse. As James Madison said in the Constitutional Convention, it was "indispensable that some provision should be made for defending the community against the incapacity, negligence, or perfidy of the chief magistrate." That is why the Founding Fathers put the impeachment provision into the Constitution. The impeachment and removal of Presidents who grossly abuse their power will have far more impact in restoring the Presidency to the reality principle than filling the White House with couches and analysts.

In saying this, the last thing I intend is to disparage psychiatry as therapy or to discourage psychiatrists from active concern with public affairs. The point is rather that each of us, politicians, historians, and psychiatrists too, must recognize the limits of this medium. Psychiatry no doubt contributes to the relief of mental problems. It is less likely to contribute to the relief of social, economic, and diplomatic problems—and these are the problems with which political leaders must deal. The reach of psychopolitics far exceeds its grasp. The notion that a democracy should empower a self-appointed group to screen its leaders is false not only to the spirit of democracy but to the psychoanalytic adventure itself.

Every psychiatrist should hang in his office, next to his

medical diploma and honorary degrees, the noble and corrosive words spoken by Thomas Mann on the seventieth birthday of Sigmund Freud:

> The analytic revelation is a revolutionary force. With it a blithe skepticism has come into the world, a mistrust which unmasks all the schemes and subterfuges of our own souls. . . . [It] inculcates the taste for understatement, as the English call it—for the deflated rather than for the inflated word, for the cult which exerts its influence by moderation, by modesty. Modesty—what a beautiful word! . . . May we hope that this may be the fundamental temper of that more blithely objective and peaceful world which the science of the unconscious may be called to usher in?

Envoi:
— • —
An Editorial
by Norman Cousins

The following brief essay is slightly modified from its initial appearance in Saturday Review*'s regular editorial space, in the issue of November 6, 1973. This was long before most of the foregoing articles or any of the three special issues were written, and as such it demonstrates Norman Cousins's long-time interest in the subject of mind research, as well as understanding of its significance.—*A.R.

From Copenhagen to Cape Town, from Chicago to Canton, from Montreal to Moscow, people appear to be caught up in the fascination with things beyond the reach of the rational intelligence. Parapsychology, extrasensory perception, and metaphysics vie as conversation pieces with theories of bioenergetic therapy, alpha waves, thought transference, breathing techniques, psychosynthesis, psychedelic therapy, meditation, Yoga, Zen Buddhism, Hare Krishna, Reichian orgone therapy, and Arica.

It would be all too easy to say we are reverting to an age of omens and incantations, but what is now happening may actually be a genuine reflection of a burgeoning interest in the untapped potentialities of human beings.

261

These popular manifestations find their counterpart in scientific probes now being made into the previously uncharted possibilities of the human mind.

The last of the great historical frontiers is now being opened up. No mysteries of outer space have been as resistant to the human brain as the way the human brain itself works and what it is. The same brain that can form questions about the riddles of macrocosm and microcosm knows very little about the process by which its own questions and contemplations are formed.

"Brain research," John C. Eccles said in a symposium several years ago on the future of the brain sciences, "is the ultimate problem confronting man. . . . This is a much bigger problem than cosmology. But for man's brain no problem would exist. The whole drama of the cosmos would be played out before empty stalls."

Neurologists, biologists, biochemists, and psychiatrists may be awed by the mysteries of the human brain, but, fortunately, they do not appear to be intimidated. Dr. Eccles has identified various fields of brain study in which research is necessary. For example, neurogenesis —how new brain cells are formed and grow and how they are converted into a communications network; neuroanatomy—now the central nervous system is connected to the brain and how it operates; neurochemistry —how the brain utilizes exotic and powerful chemicals and how these chemicals carry on vital activity inside the human system; perception—the infinitely complicated process by which neuronal activity is translated into conscious experience.

The knowledge resulting from all these studies may not be specifically directed to the present human condition, but many brain researchers agree that there is probably enough reserve capacity in the brain to meet problems far more demanding and complex than any that have so far confronted the species. The fact that most humans do not use more than 15 to 20 percent of their available intelligence would seem to indicate that the principal need is not for a better brain but for some way to make better use of the brains we have.

The concept of reserve brainpower waiting to be unlocked is comforting at a time when philosophers are asking whether the human race is smart enough to survive. The conditions of life have been running down. The dominant intelligence, however, has been trained to tribal business rather than to the operation of human society as a whole. It is possible that this challenge is related to the need for a new consciousness. It is a consciousness that can take into account the condition of the species rather than the condition of any of its subdivisions. It is a consciousness that will not be retarded by prevailing ideas.

The basic difference between a human being and the lower order of animals is that humans not only can perceive connections between causes and effects but can actually create causes that lead to desired effects. The new effect that is now needed is a planet that can be freed of the propensity for waste and desolation that has so far characterized human behavior. The kind of intelligence needed, therefore, is one that can comprehend man's place in the universal order. The process does not start at the far end; it starts with order among humans on Earth. How to create a condition of effective peace on the planet has eluded human intelligence until now; but the more we learn about the brain, the stronger is the proposition that any problem capable of being defined is capable of being solved.

Almost a century before Toynbee offered his challenge-and-response theory of history, Ludwig Gumplowicz, an Austrian philosopher, wrote that "out of friction and struggles, out of separations and unions of opposing elements, finally come forth . . . the higher cultural forms, the new civilizations, and the new unities."

New unities are now in the making. Whether they come in time will depend not on historical or anthropological laws but on the confidence human beings have in their ability to transcend old limitations. If I am right in this surmise (and I think the contents of this book now bear me out), then we may be on the verge of the most exciting period of human history.

Appendixes

APPENDIX A:

Consciousness
Research—What and Where
by John W. White

The burgeoning public interest in consciousness research is being matched by—and in part is due to—scientific and scholarly research into the nature of consciousness. The following organizations are active in some aspect of consciousness research. Many of them are open to public membership. Others publish journals and newsletters open to public subscription.

By no means should this listing be considered complete, however. Organizations researching drugs, hypnosis, biofeedback, and sleep and dreams have been deliberately omitted because they are too numerous for space requirements here. In addition, many organizations, primarily of a spiritual or religious orientation, promote research some consider as valuable as what the "hard science" approach has to offer. For information about them, consult *Spiritual Community Guide* (Spiritual Community Publications, Box 1080, San Rafael, Calif. 94920) and *International Cooperation Council Directory* (International Cooperation Council, 17819 Roscoe Blvd., Northridge, Calif. 91324).

ACADEMY OF PARAPSYCHOLOGY AND MEDICINE: 314A Second Street, Los Altos, Calif. 94022. Emphasizes parapsychological research in healing and holistic medicine. Open to public membership.

AMERICAN METAPSYCHIATRIC ASSOCIATION: 2121 North Bayshore Road, Miami, Fla. 33139. Concerned with the relation between psychiatry on the one hand, and mystical and psychic experiences on the other.

AMERICAN SOCIETY FOR PSYCHICAL RESEARCH: 5 West Seventy-third Street, New York, N.Y. 10023. An organization that performs research and conducts educational projects on the nature of psi. Open to public membership.

ASSOCIATION FOR HUMANISTIC PSYCHOLOGY: 325 Ninth Street, San Francisco, Calif. 94103. An international organization emphasizing therapy and person-centered, humanistic approaches to psychological research. Open to public membership.

ASSOCIATION FOR RESEARCH AND ENLIGHTENMENT: Box 595, Virginia Beach, Va. 23451. An association founded by the American seer Edgar Cayce for the promotion of research and the knowledge of man's spiritual nature and psychic capacities. Open to public membership.

ASSOCIATION FOR TRANSPERSONAL PSYCHOLOGY: Box 3049, Stanford, Calif. 94305. The parent organization for the newest school of psychology, transpersonal psychology. Emphasizes the higher self in people and the value of developing beyond "normality" to a transpersonal state. Open to public membership.

CALIFORNIA INSTITUTE OF TRANSPERSONAL PSYCHOLOGY: 250 Oak Grove Ave., Menlo Park, Calif. 94025. Offers a doctoral program in transpersonal psychology.

ESALEN INSTITUTE: 1793 Union Street, San Francisco, Calif. 94123. The original growth center, offering a wide range of body-mind activities for the improvement of health and the expansion of awareness.

FOUNDATION FOR MIND RESEARCH: Box 600, Pomona, N.Y. 10970. A foundation that studies altered states of consciousness, accelerated learning, the psychology of the creative process, the induction of religious-type experiences, and other aspects of higher consciousness.

FOUNDATION FOR RESEARCH ON THE NATURE OF MAN: 402 Buchanan Blvd., Durham, N.C. 27708. A foundation set up by J. B. Rhine for parapsychological research.

HIGHER SENSE PERCEPTION RESEARCH FOUNDATION: 8668½ Wilshire Blvd., Beverly Hills, Calif. 90211. A foundation that studies the energies underlying psychic perception.

HUMAN DIMENSIONS INSTITUTE: 4380 Main Street, Buffalo, N.Y. 14226. Offers a wide-ranging program of studies in human potential.

INSTITUTE FOR CONSCIOUSNESS AND MUSIC: 721 St. John's Road, Baltimore, Md. 21210. Conducts research and growth activities emphasizing creativity through music.

INSTITUTE FOR THE STUDY OF CONSCIOUSNESS: 2924 Benvenue Ave., Berkeley, Calif. 94705. An institute that conducts research and educational activities on the nature of consciousness.

INSTITUTE OF NOETIC SCIENCES: 530 Oak Grove Ave., Menlo Park, Calif. 94025. Sponsors research, educational, consulting, and public-information activities about the nature of consciousness and the mind-body relation. Open to public membership.

JOHNSTON COLLEGE: Program for Transpersonal Education, University of Redlands, Redlands, Calif. 92373. Offers bachelor's and master's degrees in transpersonal psychology.

KUNDALINI RESEARCH FOUNDATION: 10 East Thirty-ninth Street, New York, N.Y. 10016. A foundation that sponsors research and public-information activities about the nature of *kundalini,* the evolutionary energy underlying mental faculties, spiritual experience, and higher consciousness, as described by Gopi Krishna.

MAIMONIDES MEDICAL CENTER: Division of Parapsychology and Psychophysics, 4802 Tenth Ave., Brooklyn, N.Y. 11219. Conducts psychic research with emphasis on altered states of consciousness.

MANKIND RESEARCH UNLIMITED: 1325½ Wisconsin Ave., Washington, D.C. 20007. An organization that conducts research, educational, and public-information activities concerning a wide range of psychic, paraphysical, and mind-body phenomena.

NEW YORK UNIVERSITY SCHOOL OF CONTINUING EDUCATION: 2 University Place, New York, N.Y. 10003. Offers programs in mind research.

PARAPSYCHOLOGY FOUNDATION: 29 West Fifty-seventh Street, New York, N.Y. 10019. A foundation that sponsors research, educational, and public-information activities in parapsychology.

PSYCHICAL RESEARCH FOUNDATION: Duke Station, Durham, N.C. 27706. A foundation that conducts research and public-information activities concerning the question of life after death. Open to public membership.

PSYCHOSYNTHESIS INSTITUTE: 150 Doherty Way, Redwood City, Calif. 94062. An institute that promotes the approach to higher mind-body potential called psychosynthesis, developed by Roberto Assagioli.

R. M. BUCKE MEMORIAL SOCIETY: 4453 Maisonneuve Blvd. West, Montreal, 215, Canada. Continues the tradition of R. M. Bucke, author of *Cosmic Consciousness*, by exploring states of mystical illumination and all forms of human experience that seem of "absolute" or "ultimate" significance to the individual.

SPIRITUAL FRONTIERS FELLOWSHIP: Executive Plaza, 10715 Winner Road, Independence, Mo. 64052. An organization that conducts research, educational, and public-information activities about the spiritual-psychic nature of man as recorded in the Bible. Open to public membership.

STANFORD RESEARCH INSTITUTE: 333 Ravenswood

Ave., Menlo Park, Calif. 94025. Conducts scientific and scholarly research into the nature of human consciousness.

Students International Meditation Society: 1015 Gayley Ave., Los Angeles, Calif. 90024. The national headquarters for the transcendental meditation movement and a major clearinghouse for meditation-research information.

University of Virginia: Division of Parapsychology, Department of Psychiatry, School of Medicine, Charlottesville, Va. 22901. Psychic research, with current emphasis on out-of-the-body experience, reincarnation, and life after death.

In addition to the organizations and universities cited above, various colleges and universities offer study programs in consciousness research and conduct scientific and scholarly research.

California Institute of Asian Studies: 3494 Twenty-first Street, San Francisco, Calif. 94110. The institute offers a doctoral program in transpersonal and integral psychology.

California School of Professional Studies: 480 Potrero Ave., San Francisco, Calif. 94110. Offers a doctoral program in psychology that includes transpersonal courses and the possibility of transpersonal-dissertation research.

City College of the City of New York: Department of Psychology, New York, N.Y. 10031. Offers supervised work in parapsychology at the undergraduate, master's, and doctoral levels for degrees in psychology.

College of Oriental Studies: 939 S. New Hampshire, Los Angeles, Calif. 90006. Offers bachelor, master's, and doctoral programs in Oriental studies, Buddhist philosophy, Zen studies, comparative religion, and philosophy.

Humanistic Psychology Institute: 325 Ninth

Street, San Francisco, Calif. 94103. Offers doctoral programs in parapsychology and nondegree courses in parapsychology leading to a doctoral degree in psychology.

INSTITUTE OF MYSTICAL AND PARAPSYCHOLOGICAL STUDIES: John F. Kennedy University, 1124 Ferry Street, Martinez, Calif. 94553. Offers bachelor's and master's degrees with a concentration in mysticism and parapsychology.

PSYCHOLOGICAL STUDIES INSTITUTE: 580 College Ave., Palo Alto, Calif. 93404. Offers a doctoral program emphasizing integrative psychology—Eastern, existential, and humanistic.

UNIVERSITY OF CALIFORNIA, DAVIS: Department of Psychology, Davis, Calif. 95616. Offers supervised work leading to a doctoral degree in psychology.

UNIVERSITY OF CALIFORNIA, SANTA CRUZ: Graduate Office, Santa Cruz, Calif. 95064. Offers a doctoral program in the history of consciousness.

UNIVERSITY OF THE TREES: Box 644, Boulder Creek, Calif. 95006. Offers a three-year course in meditation and conducts research into radiational paraphysics and the nature of consciousness.

WEST GEORGIA COLLEGE: Carrolton, Ga. 30117. Offers undergraduate and master's programs with emphasis on humanistic and transpersonal psychology.

APPENDIX B:
A Sampler of Recent Books
1973-1976

To prepare anything like a complete bibliography of the major subject areas covered here would require a much fatter volume than this one. From the sagging bookshelves full of material available, we have arbitrarily decided to stick to a scattering of books published from 1973 to 1976—on occasion including an older book that emerged during that period in a revised edition (in which case it is so noted). It is absolutely inevitable that we will have left out somebody's favorite book in one area or another.

Drawing the line at 1973 meant omitting such books as *The History of Psychiatry* by Franz Alexander and Sheldon T. Selesnick, Nigel Calder's *The Mind of Man,* Isaac Asimov's *The Human Brain,* Moshe Feldenkrais's *Awareness Through Movement,* as well as *Mind Games* and *The Varieties of Psychedelic Experience,* co-authored by Jean Houston and Robert Masters. It meant listing Carlos Castaneda's *Tales of Power,* but not his earlier books in the don Juan series; Joseph Chilton Pearce's *Exploring the Crack in the Cosmic Egg,* but not the original *The Crack in the Cosmic Egg.* We could not include Charles Tart's *Al-*

tered States of Consciousness, but have listed his later *States of Consciousness.* And so on.

We have refrained from attempting evaluations of the books listed, but cannot resist expressing our admiration for Silvano Arieti's now-classic six-volume *Handbook of Psychiatry;* and, among the self-help books in psychiatry, to express our preference for the Park-Shapiro book, *You Are Not Alone.*

This bibliography, in a word, is suggestive rather than exhaustive or definitive.

MIND AND CONSCIOUSNESS (GENERAL)

Drug Abuse Council, *Altered States of Consciousness: Current Views and Research Problems,* Washington, D.C.

Ferguson, Marilyn, *The Brain Revolution: The Frontiers of Mind Research,* Taplinger, New York.

Lee, Phillip R., et al., *Symposium on Consciousness,* The Viking Press, New York.

Ornstein, Robert E., *The Mind Field,* Grossman (The Viking Press), New York.

———, *The Nature of Human Consciousness,* The Viking Press, New York.

Smith, Adam, *Powers of Mind,* Random House, New York.

Tart, Charles, *States of Consciousness,* E. P. Dutton, New York.

White, John (ed.), *Frontiers of Consciousness: The Meeting Ground Between Inner and Outer Reality,* Julian Press, New York.

PSI

Castaneda, Carlos, *Tales of Power,* Simon & Schuster, New York.

Geller, Uri, *My Story,* Praeger, New York.

Krippner, Stanley, and Rubin, Daniel (eds.), *The Kirlian Aura: Photographing the Galaxies of Life,* Anchor/Doubleday, Garden City, N.Y.

LeShan, Lawrence, *The Medium, the Mystic, and the Physicist: Toward a General Theory of the Paranormal,* The Viking Press, New York.

Mitchell, Edgar D., *Psychic Exploration: A Challenge for Science,* G. P. Putnam's Sons, New York.

Moss, Thelma, *The Probability of the Impossible,* J.P. Tarcher, Los Angeles.

Ostrander, Sheila, and Schroeder, Lynn, *Handbook of PSI Discoveries,* G. P. Putnam's Sons, New York.

Panati, Charles, *Supersenses: Our Potential for Parasensory Experience,* Quadrangle, New York.

Puharich, Andrija, *Uri: A Journal of the Mystery of Uri Geller,* Bantam Books, New York.

Randall, John L., *Parapsychology and the Nature of Life,* Harper & Row, New York.

Regush, June and Nicholas, *PSI: The Other World Catalogue,* G. P. Putnam's Sons, New York.

Targ, Russell, and Puthoff, Harold, *Mind-Reach: Scientists Look at Psychic Ability,* Delacorte Press, New York.

Taylor, John, *Superminds: A Scientist Looks at the Paranormal,* The Viking Press, New York.

Watson, Lyall, *Supernature,* Anchor/Doubleday, Garden City, N.Y.

BIOFEEDBACK

Brown, Barbara B., *New Mind, New Body—Biofeedback: New Directions for the Mind,* Harper & Row, New York.

Birk, Lee, *Behavioral Medicine: The Clinical Uses of Biofeedback,* Grune, New York.

Jonas, Gerald, *Visceral Learning,* Cornerstone, New York.

Zaffuto, Anthony A. and Mary Q., *Alphagenics: How to Use Your Brain Waves to Improve Your Life,* Doubleday, New York.

DREAMS

Faraday, Ann, *The Dream Game,* Harper & Row, New York.

Garfield, Patricia, *Creative Dreaming,* Simon & Schuster, New York.

Jones, Richard M., *The New Psychology of Dreaming,* The Viking Press, New York.

Ullman, Montague, Krippner, Stanley, with Vaughan, Alan, *Dream Telepathy: Scientific Experiments in the Supernatural,* Macmillan, New York.

Woods, Ralph L., and Greenhouse, Herbert B. (eds.), *The New World of Dreams,* Macmillan, New York.

HEALING

Boyd, Doug, *Rolling Thunder,* Random House, New York.

Dooley, Anne, *Every Wall a Door,* E. P. Dutton, New York.

Kiev, Ari, *Magic, Faith and Healing,* The Free Press, New York.

Kruger, Helen, *Other Healers, Other Cures,* Bobbs-Merrill, New York.

Nolen, William A., *Healing: A Doctor in Search of a Miracle,* Random House, New York.

St. Clair, David, *Psychic Healing,* Doubleday, New York.

MEDITATION AND YOGA

Benson, Herbert, *The Relaxation Response,* William Morrow, New York.

Bloomfield, Harold H., Cain, Michael P., et al., *TM: Discovering Inner Energy and Overcoming Stress,* Dell, New York.

Denniston, Denise, and McWilliams, Peter, *The TM Book,* Warner Books, New York.

Forem, Jack, *Transcendental Meditation,* E. P. Dutton, New York.

LeShan, Lawrence, *How to Meditate: A Guide to Self-Discovery,* Little, Brown, Boston.

Satprem, *Sri Aurobindo, or the Adventure of Consciousness,* Harper & Row, New York.

Segesman, Margrit, *Wings of Power,* Harper & Row, New York.

White, John (ed.), *What Is Meditation?* Anchor/Double-day, Garden City, N.Y.

Miscellaneous (Mind and Consciousness)

Gallwey, W. Timothy, *The Inner Game of Tennis,* Random House, New York.

Grof, Stanislov, *Realms of the Human Unconscious: Observations from LSD Research,* The Viking Press, New York.

Jaynes, Julius, *The Origins of Consciousness in the Breakdown of the Bicameral Mind,* Houghton Mifflin, Boston.

Leonard, George, *The Ultimate Athlete: Re-Visioning Sports, Physical Education, and the Body,* The Viking Press, New York.

Naranjo, Claudio, *The Healing Journey: New Approaches to Consciousness,* Pantheon, New York.

Pearce, Joseph C., *Exploring the Crack in the Cosmic Egg: Split Minds and Meta-Realities,* Julian Press, New York.

The Brain and Neuroscience

Eccles, John C., *The Understanding of the Brain,* McGraw-Hill, New York.

Gardner, Howard, *The Shattered Mind,* Alfred A. Knopf, New York.

Gaylin, Willard M., Meister, Joel S., and Neville, Robert C., *Operating on the Mind,* Basic Books, New York.

Hart, Leslie A., *How the Brain Works: A New Understanding of Human Learning, Emotion, and Thinking,* Basic Books, New York.

Luria, A. R., *The Working Brain: An Introduction to Neuropsychology,* Basic Books, New York.

Penfield, Wilder, *The Mystery of Mind: A Critical Study of Consciousness and the Human Brain,* Princeton University Press, Princeton, N.J.

Pines, Maya, *The Brain Changers: Scientists and the New Mind Control,* Harcourt Brace Jovanovich, New York.

Pool, J. Lawrence, *Your Brain and Nerves,* Charles Scribner's Sons, New York.

Rose, Steven, *The Conscious Brain,* Alfred A. Knopf, New York.

PSYCHIATRY AND PSYCHOANALYSIS (GENERAL)

Arieti, Silvano, *American Handbook of Psychiatry* (6 vols.), Basic Books, New York (revised ed.).

Boothe, Bert E., Rosenfeld, Anne H., and Walker, Edward L., *Toward a Science of Psychiatry: Impact of the Research Development Program of the National Institute of Mental Health,* Brooks/Cole (John Wiley), New York.

Coles, Robert, *The Mind's Fate: Ways of Seeing Psychiatry and Psychoanalysis,* Atlantic Monthly Press (Little, Brown), Boston.

Collier, Herbert L., *What's Psychotherapy and Who Needs It?,* O'Sullivan, Woodside & Co., Phoenix.

Freedman, Alfred M., Kaplan, Harold I., and Sadock, Benjamin J., *Comprehensive Textbook of Psychiatry* (2 vols.), Williams & Wilkins, Baltimore.

Fromm-Reichmann, Frieda, *Psychoanalysis and Psychotherapy: Selected Papers,* University of Chicago Press, Chicago (revised ed.).

Harper, Robert A., *Psychoanalysis and Psychotherapy: 36 Systems,* Jason Aronson, New York.

Howells, John G., (ed.), *World History of Psychiatry,* Brunner/Mazel, New York.

Kahn, Samuel, *Essays in Freudian Psychoanalysis,* Philosophical Library, New York.

Klein, Melanie, *Love, Guilt and Reparation & Other Works, 1921–1945,* Delacorte Press, New York.

———, *Envy and Gratitude & Other Works, 1946–1963,* Delacorte Press, New York.

Klopfer, Walter G., and Reed, Max R. (eds.), *Problems in Psychotherapy: An Eclectic Approach,* Hemisphere (John Wiley), New York.

Kovel, Joel, *A Complete Guide to Therapy: From Psychoanalysis to Behavior Modification,* Pantheon, New York.

Milt, Harry, *Basic Handbook of Mental Illness*, Charles Scribner's Sons, New York.

Rees, W. L. Linford, *A Short Textbook of Psychiatry*, The English Universities Press, London.

Robins, Eli, *Psychiatry 1975*, (*Medical World News*), McGraw-Hill, New York.

Tennov, Dorothy, *Psychotherapy: The Hazardous Cure*, Anchor/Doubleday, Garden City, N.Y.

Weiner, I. B., *Principles of Psychotherapy*, John Wiley, New York.

Yap, P. M., *Comparative Psychiatry: A Theoretical Framework*, University of Toronto Press, Toronto.

The New Psychotherapies

Bassin, Alexander et al. (eds.), *The Reality Therapy Reader: A Survey of the Work of William Glasser*, Harper & Row, New York.

Beck, Aaron T., *Cognitive Therapy and the Emotional Disorders*, International Universities Press, New York.

Bloom, Bernard L., *Changing Patterns of Psychiatric Care*, Behavior Publications, New York.

Bry, Adelaide, *est: 60 Hours That Transform Your Life*, Harper & Row, New York.

Frederick, Carl, *est: Playing the Game the New Way*, Delacorte Press, New York.

Greenwald, Harold (ed.), *Active Psychotherapy*, Jason Aronson, New York.

Harper, Robert A., *The New Psychotherapies*, Prentice-Hall, Englewood Cliffs, N.J.

Hilts, Philip J., *Behavior Mod*, Harper's Magazine Press, New York.

Janov, Arthur, and Holden, E. Michael, *Primal Man: The New Consciousness*, Thomas Y. Crowell, New York.

Reynolds, David K., *Morita Psychotherapy*, University of California Press, Berkeley.

Rhinehart, Luke, *The Book of est*, Holt, Rinehart and Winston, New York.

Rogers, Carl, *Carl Rogers on Encounter Groups,* Harrow Books (Harper & Row), New York.

Rosenblatt, Daniel, *Opening Doors: What Happens in Gestalt Therapy,* Harper & Row, New York.

Segal, Julius (editor-in-chief), *Research in the Service of Mental Health: Report of the Research Task Force of the National Institute of Mental Health,* National Institute of Mental Health, Rockville, Md.

Weiner, Melvin L., *The Cognitive Unconscious: A Piagetian Approach to Psychotherapy,* International Psychological Press, New York.

SCHIZOPHRENIA

Arieti, Silvano, *Interpretation of Schizophrenia,* Basic Books, New York (revised ed.).

Cancro, Robert, Fox, Norma, and Shapiro, Lester (eds.), *Strategic Intervention in Schizophrenia: Current Developments in Treatment,* Behavior Publications, New York.

Whitehorn, John C., and Betz, Barbara, *Effective Psychotherapy with the Schizophrenic Patient,* Jason Aronson, New York.

Wolf, Stewart and Berle, Beatrice B. (eds.), *The Biology of the Schizophrenic Process,* Plenum Press, New York.

DEPRESSION

Becker, Joseph, *Depression: Theory and Research,* V. H. Winston & Sons, Washington.

Flach, Frederic F., *The Secret Strength of Depression,* J. B. Lippincott, New York.

_____, and Draghi, Suzanne C. (eds.), *The Nature and Treatment of Depression,* John Wiley & Sons, New York.

Friedman, Raymond J., and Katz, Martin M. (eds.), *The Psychology of Depression: Contemporary Theory and Research,* Halsted/Wiley, New York.

Kline, Nathan S., *From Sad to Glad: Kline on Depression,* G. P. Putnam's Sons, New York.

Knauth, Percy, *A Season in Hell,* Harper & Row, New York.

Lesse, Stanley (ed.), *Masked Depression,* Jason Aronson, New York.

Levitt, Eugene E., and Lubin, Bernard, *Depression: Concepts, Controversies, and Some New Facts,* Springer Publishing Co., New York.

Seligman, Martin E. P., *Helplessness: On Depression, Development and Death,* Scientific American Books, W. H. Freeman & Co., San Francisco.

Biology and Pharmacology (Mental Illness)

Ayd, Frank J., Jr. (ed.), *Rational Psychopharmacotherapy and the Right to Treatment,* Ayd Medical Communications, Baltimore.

Denber, Herman C. B. (ed.), *Psychopharmacological Treatment: Theory and Practice,* Marcel Dekker, New York.

de Ropp, Robert S., *Drugs and the Mind,* Delacorte Press/ Seymour Lawrence, New York (revised ed.).

Fieve, Ronald R., *Moodswing: The Third Revolution in Psychiatry,* William Morrow, New York.

Fink, Max, Kety, Seymour, et al. (eds.), *Psychobiology of Convulsive Therapy,* V. H. Winston & Sons, Washington.

Goodman, Louis S., and Gilman, Alfred G. (eds.), *The Pharmacological Basis of Therapeutics,* Macmillan, New York (5th ed.).

Iversen, S., and Iversen, L., *Behavioral Pharmacology,* Oxford University Press, New York.

Kiev, Ari (ed.), *Somatic Manifestations of Depressive Disorders,* Excerpta Medica, Amsterdam.

Mendels, Joseph (ed.), *Biological Psychiatry,* John Wiley & Sons, New York.

Snyder, Solomon, *Madness and the Brain,* McGraw-Hill, New York.

Swazey, Judith P., *Chlorpromazine in Psychiatry: A Study of Therapeutic Innovation,* M.I.T. Press, Cambridge, Mass.

Nutrition and Mental Health

Cheraskin, E., and Ringsdorf, W. M., Jr., with Brecher, Arline, *Psychodietetics,* Stein & Day, New York.

Fried, John J., *The Vitamin Conspiracy,* Saturday Review Press (E. P. Dutton), New York.

Passwater, Richard, *Supernutrition,* The Dial Press, New York.

Pfeiffer, Carl, and the staff of the Brain Bio Center, *Mental and Elemental Nutrients,* Keats, New Canaan, Conn.

The Antipsychiatry Movement

Boyers, Robert (ed.), *R. D. Laing & Anti-Psychiatry,* Farrar, Straus & Giroux, New York.

Szasz, Thomas, *The Myth of Mental Illness,* Harper & Row, New York (revised ed.).

Torrey, Fuller E., *The Death of Psychiatry,* Chilton, Radnor, Pa.

Self-Help

Andreasen, Nancy C., *Understanding Mental Illness: A Layman's Guide,* Augsburg Publishing House, Minneapolis.

Herman, Melvin, and Freeman, Lucy, *The Pursuit of Mental Health,* Macmillan, New York.

Park, Clara C., with Shapiro, Leon N., *You Are Not Alone: Understanding and Dealing with Mental Illness; a Guide for Patients, Families, Doctors and Other Professionals,* Atlantic Monthly Press (Little, Brown), Boston.

Torrey, Fuller E., *Why Did You Do That?: Shrink Yourself,* Chilton, Radnor, Pa.

Miscellaneous (Psychotherapy)

Abel, Theodora M., and Métraux, Rhoda, *Culture and Psychotherapy,* College and University Press, New Haven, Conn.

Becker, Ernest, *Revolution in Psychiatry,* The Free Press, New York.

Benziger, Barbara F., *Speaking Out: Therapists and Patients —How They Cure and Cope with Mental Illness Today,* Walker & Co., New York.

Bromberg, Walter, *From Shaman to Psychotherapist: A History of the Treatment of Mental Illness,* Henry Regnery Co., Chicago.

Crocetti, Guido M., Spiro, Herzel R., and Siassi, Iradj, *Contemporary Attitudes Toward Mental Illness,* University of Pittsburgh Press, Pittsburgh.

Dean, Stanley R. (ed.), *Psychiatry and Mysticism,* Nelson-Hall, Chicago.

Donaldson, Kenneth, *Insanity Inside Out,* Crown, New York.

Fincher, Jack, *Human Intelligence,* G. P. Putnam's Sons, New York.

Fischer, Joel, and Gochros, Harvey L., *Planned Behavior Change: Behavior Modification in Social Work,* The Free Press, New York.

Fornari, Franco, *The Psychoanalysis of War,* Anchor/Doubleday, Garden City, N.Y.

Frankl, Viktor E., *The Unconscious God: Psychotherapy and Theology,* Simon & Schuster, New York.

Lifton, Robert Jay, *The Life of the Self: Toward a New Psychology,* Simon & Schuster, New York.

————, with Eric Olson (eds.), *Explorations in Psychohistory: The Wellfleet Papers,* Simon & Schuster, New York.

Orlinsky, David E., and Howard, Kenneth I., *Varieties of Psychotherapeutic Experience: Multivariate Analyses of Patients' and Therapists' Reports,* Teachers College Press, New York.

Siegler, Miriam, and Osmond, Humphrey, *Models of Madness, Models of Medicine,* Macmillan, New York.

Welford, A. T. (ed.), *Man Under Stress,* John Wiley, New York.

Williams, Elizabeth F., *Notes of a Feminist Therapist,* Praeger, New York.

Index

Accelerated mental process
(AMP), 16–17
ACTH hormone, 95–96
Acupuncture, 54
Adler, Alfred, xi
Aggression, and brain stimulation, 105–106
Agranoff, Bernard, 92–93
Albert, Martin, 121
Alcoholic blackout, compared to fragmentary amnesia, 99–100
Alcoholism, and diet, 234–235
Alexander, F. Matthias, 16, 50
Alexander, Franz G., 178
Alexander technique, 50
Alexia, 122
All-India Institute of Medical Sciences, 53
Altered states of consciousness (ASC), 4, 20, 48
and linear time, 15–17
Altered States of Consciousness Induction Device (ASCID), 22
American Presidency:
accountability, 256–257
and mental illness, 246–260

restoring to reality, 256–259
Amnesia, alcohol-induced, 98–100
Amphetamine, 88–89, 223–224
Amygdala, 87
signals of, 107
Anderson, Poul, 69
Androids, 67
Andy, O.J., 149–150
Annis, Robert, 142
Anxiety, and biofeedback, 38–39
Aphasia, 114
therapy for, 121
and visual artistry, 118
Apparitions of the dead, 60
Apparitions of the living, 60
Arasteh, A. Reza, 53
Arica training, 188
Arieti, Silvano, 243
Asimov, Isaac, 62–74
Assagioli, Roberto, 188
Austin, James H., 133–136
Autogenic training, 50
Avery, Roger, 164
Axelrod, Julius, 219

Backster, Cleve, 53, 54
Ban, Thomas, 229–230

Barlow, Horace, 141
Basmajian, John, 36, 44
Behavior modification, 157, 193
Behavior therapy, 185–186
Behaviorism, 127–128
Benford, Gregory, 73
Berkeley, George, 145
Berne, Eric, 189
Bester, Alfred, 71
Bickford, Reginald, 163
Bioenergetics, 50
Biofeedback, 34–46, 48–49, 185–
    186, 193–194
  future of, 46
  and heartbeat rate, 37
  meaning of, 35–36
  practical applications of, 45–
    46
  and sensory information, 40–
    41
  and structural capabilities of
    body, 43–44
  and tension and anxiety, 38–
    39
Biological clock, 106
Blakemore, Colin, 139–142
Blish, James, 73
Bock, Darrell, 130
Body:
  involuntary functions of, 35
  muscle tension, 38–39
  voluntary control, 40, 42–43
Body consciousness, 49–50
Body-mind relation, 27–33
  see also Mind-body relation
Bogen, Joseph, 125
Boulle, Pierre, 67
Bova, Ben, 62–74
Brain:
  cerebellum, 84
  cerebral cortex, 83
  conscious and unconscious,
    78–79
  electrical and chemical stimu-
    lation of, 101–111

and environment, 110–111
  guide to structure and func-
    tion of, 82–87
  hemispheres of, 124–133
  hypothalamus, 87
  informational capacity, 10–11
  left-right dominance, 128–130
  limbic system, 152–154
  lobes of, 83
  and nutrition, 111, 232–235
  overview, 77–81
  pacemakers for, 162–173
  physical manipulation of, 79–
    81
  psychochemistry of, 88–89
Brain, Russell, x
Brain damage, 112–123
  cerebral vascular accident
    (stroke), 113
  in child vs. adult, 122
  Korsakoff's disease, 116–118
  and relationships among abili-
    ties, 115
  selectivity of, 114
Brainwashing, 80
Brain-wave control, 49
Brown, Barbara, 34–46, 49
Brown, Norman O., 53
Bullitt, William C., 255
Bunney, William, 235

Campbell, John W., Jr., 64, 71,
    72
Čapek, Karel, 67
Carlsson, Arvid, 223
Castaneda, Carlos, xiii–xiv, 5, 55,
    147
Castration anxiety, 207
Center for Preventive Psychiatry
    (CPP), 211
Central nervous system, 83–84
Cerebellar stimulator, 162–173
Cerebral allergies, 234
Cerebral hemispheres, domi-
    nance of, 128–130

Cerebral hemispheres *(cont'd)*
and eye movements, 133–136
Chemitrodes, 109
Cheraskin, E., 229
Children:
hyperactive, 150, 234
and preventive psychiatry,
212–213
Chisholm, Brock, 249
Chlorpromazine, 222
Chomsky, Noam, 51
Clairsentience, 59
Clairvoyance, 59
Clark, Kenneth, 251–252, 255
Clarke, Arthur C., 7
Clifford, Clark, 247
Conflict, realistic and nonrealistic, 249
Consciousness:
altered states of, 4, 20, 48
and brain mechanism, 131–133
crisis of, 19
as cure, 201
overview, 3–6
need for new, 263
research areas, 48–57
research organizations, list of,
267–272
revolution of, 47–57
science of (noetics), 47–48
Computers, 7–9
and science fiction, 68–69
Computer Assisted Dialogue
(CAD), 7
Cooper, Graham, 140
Cooper, Irving, 108, 162–173
Corpus callosum, 124–125
Cousins, Norman, xi, 261–264
Creativity, 22–23, 118–119
Freud on, 254–255
and manic depression, 244
Crisis intervention, 213
Cross-sensing, 24
Cryosurgery, 165–167

CSB (chemical stimulation of the
brain), 109
and inhibition of pain, 109–110
Cultural trance, 19, 21
Cyborg, 8

Dabrowsky, Kascimerz, 53
Darwin, Charles, 64
Davis, Adelle, 229, 230, 233
Dean, Stanley, 52
Death, process of, 56
de Camp, L. Sprague, 70, 72
Decision making, 41
and conscious mind, 132–133
Defeudis, Francis, 110
Delaney, Samuel R., 69
Delgado, José, xii, 101–111
recent research findings, 103
del Rey, Lester, 68, 69
Dematerialization, 59
Depression:
chemical treatment for, 237–245
diagnosis of, 241–242
and neurotransmitters, 219–220
orthodox treatment for, 240
symptoms of, 238
unipolar and bipolar, 240–241
Descartes, René, x
Dewey, John, 16
DeWied, David, 95, 98
Drugs:
antidepressant, 240
antihistaminic, 221–222
chlorpromazine, 88
effects on mood, 219–220
hallucinogenic, 221
L-Dopa, 166
lithium, 220–221, 240, 244–245
and memory, 92–100
neurochemistry of addiction,
110

Drugs *(cont'd)*
  tranquilizers, 154
Dynamic unconsciousness, 201
Dyrud, Jarl, 180, 199–210
Dyslexia, 122, 123
Dystonia musculorum deformans, 165, 167–169

Eccles, John C., 262
Edgar, Harold, 155, 157
Education, and cerebral hemispheres, 130–131
Eidetic perception, 21
Elderly, the:
  and memory, 94–95, 96
  and sensory acuity, 24
Electroconvulsive shock, and memory, 94, 95–96
Electroencephalogram (EEG), 85
Elkes, Joel, 17n, 180
Endorphins, xv
Engelhardt, H. Tristram, Jr., x
Engrams, 91
Environment:
  effect on brain, 110–111
  and musical talent, 143–144
  and psychiatry, 196–198
  and vision, 137
Epilepsy, 163
  and corpus callosum removal, 124
  and ESB, 108, 154, 160, 171
Erhard Seminars Training *(est)*, 191–192
Erikson, Erik, 207
ESB (electrical stimulation of the brain), 102–108, 159–161
Ethics:
  "informed consent," 155–157, 169–171
  of neurosurgery, 167–168
Ewald, J., 103
Exobiology, 50–51
Extrapyramidal system, 87

Extrasensory perception (ESP), 58, 59
Extraterrestrial intelligence, 71–74
Eye:
  light detection ability of, 9–10
  movements, and cerebral hemispheres, 133–136

Family therapy, 190
Feature extraction, 87
Feingold, Ben, 234
Feis, Herbert, 248, 255
Feldenkrais, Moshe, 16, 30, 50
Feldenkrais method, 50
Feminist therapy, 190–191
Fieve, Ronald R., 239–245
Fink, Max, 96
Foundation for Mind Research (FMR), 15–26, 29–32
Frank, Jerome D., 194
Fredericks, Carlton, 234
Free association, 203
Freeman, John, 235
Freeman, Walter, 151–152
Freud, Sigmund, 178, 199–202, 205–206, 207–208, 240, 248, 251, 254–255
Frontal-lobe syndrome, 152
Frost, Barrie, 142
Fulton, James, 151
Fulton, John, 104
Futurism, 7–9, 13

Gardner, Howard, 112–123
Garrett, Randall, 70
Geller, Uri, 54
General extrasensory perception (GESP), 59
Genes:
  and cerebral dominance, 129
  informational capacity, 10
Gibson, Robert, 235
Gold, Paul E., 97
Goodwin, Donald W., 99

Green, Elmer, 49
Greenwald, Harold, 179
Group psychotherapy, 189–190
Gumplowicz, Ludwig, 263

Halliday, Michael, 51
Halpern, Charles, 156
Hamilton, Edmond, 64–65, 68
Handbook of Psychiatry (Arieti), 274
Handedness, 128–130
Hauntings of the dead, 60
Hawkins, David, 229, 230, 233, 234
Heath, Robert, 108, 160
Heinlein, Robert A., 69, 70, 72
Heisenberg, Werner, 101
Helm, Nancy, 121
Hendin, David, 162–173
Herbert, Frank, 66
Heredity vs. environment controversy, xii
    in schizophrenia, 225–226
Hess, Walter, 103
Hieronymus, T.G., 54
Hirsch, Helmut, 140
The History of Psychiatry (Alexander and Selesnick), 178
Hoffer, Abram, 231–232, 233
Homans, George, 201
Houston, Jean, 15–26, 48, 55
Hoyle, Fred, 73
Hubel, David, 138–139, 141
Human potential:
    and material sacrifice, 14
    psychenaut program, 17–26
    under study, 22–26
    waste of, 11–12
Human potential movement, *see* Psi movement
Humanistic therapy, 186–187
Hutschnecker, Arnold A., 252–253, 255
Hyperresponsive Syndrome, 149–150

Hypoglycemia, 234
Hypothalamus, 87

Ichazo, Oscar, 188
ICSS (intracranial self-stimulation), 160
Ideomotor reflex, 16
Image thinking, 22–23
Imagination, as mind-body visualization, 16
In a Darkness (Wechsler), 253
Individuality, 129–130
Institute of Noetic Sciences, 48
Intellect, and cerebral hemispheres, 129–130
Intelligence, manufactured, 65–66
Intronaut, 17n
Iproniazid, 219–220
Isgur, Jay, 123

James, Daniel B., 68
James, William, 55, 58
Janov, Arthur, 192–193
Jefferson, Thomas, 256
Johnson, Lyndon, 257

Kahn, Herman, 7
Kamiya, Joe, 49
Katz, Bernard, 219
Kaufman, Bernard T., 233
Kennedy, Edward, 157
Kety, Seymour S., 180, 215–226, 235
Keyes, Daniel, 66
Kiev, Ari, 195–198
Kirlian photography, 54
Kliman, Ann, 213
Kliman, Gilbert W., 211
Kline, Nathan S., 105, 239–245
Klivington, Kenneth A., 77–81, 82–87
Knight, Frank, 203
Knowledge, as evil, 63–64
Kolakowski, Donald, 130

Korsakoff's disease, 116–118
Krishna, Gopi, 53
Kubler-Ross, Elizabeth, 56
Kuhn, Thomas, 55
Kundalini, 53

Laborit, Henri-Marie, 222
Laing, R.D., xiii, 52, 179
Lamb, Sydney, 51
Language:
  and creativity, 118–119
  and thought, 119–120
Lashley, Karl, 91–92, 93
Lazarus, Arnold, 199–200
L-Dopa, 166, 223
Learning:
  how to learn, 144
  and sensitive periods, 143
Learning disabilities, 122–123
Lee, Russel V., 250–251, 252, 255
Leonard, George, xiv, 7–14
Levitation, 60
Levy, Jerry, 129
Lewin, Roger, 137–144
Lilly, John, 52
Limbic system, 87, 152–154
Linguistics, 51
  cognitive, 51
  language acquisition, 143
  stratificational grammar, 51
  systemic grammar, 51
  transformational grammar, 51
Lipton, Morris, 229
Lithium, 220–221, 240, 244–245
  failure to prescribe, 242
Lobotomy, 151–152
Locke, John, 145
Luria, A.R., 97–98

Madison, James, 259
Malleus Maleficarum, 177–178
Mandell, Marshall, 233
Mania, and neurotransmitters, 220–221
Manic depression, 244–245

Mann, Thomas, 260
Mark, Vernon, 156–157
Marmor, Judd, 254
Martial arts, 49
Maslow, Abraham, 56, 187
Masters, Robert, 27–33, 55
Materialization, 59
"Mauve" factor, 231–232
McCaffrey, Anne, 68
McGaugh, James, 91, 93–94, 97
Meaning, web of, 204–205
Meditation research, 51–52
Mediumship, 60
Melancholy, *see* Depression
Memory, 90–100
  and aging, 90–91, 94–95, 96
  chemical aspect of, 92–100
  perfect, danger of, 97–98
  stages of, 92–93
  two forms of, 117–118
Menninger, Karl, 255
Mental hospitals, 177–178
Mental illness:
  biochemistry of, 215–226
  chemical theory of, 79–80
  genetic factors, 224–226
Metalinguistics, 51
Metanoia, 52
Metapsychiatry, 52–53
Metapsychology, 205–206
Mind:
  concept of, ix–x
  new awareness concerning, 44–45
  science of, and traditional science, 4–6, 9, 34–35, 41–42, 44–45, 203–205
Mind-body relation, 18, 42
  training of, 20–21
  see also Body-mind relation
Mind control, 80–81
Mind expansion, *see* Altered states of consciousness
Mind research:
  bibliography, 273–283

Mind research *(cont'd)*
  overview, 261–264
Minority groups, and psychiatry, 196–197
Mitchell, Don, 141
Mitchell, Edgar D., 48
Moniz, Egas, 151
Monoamine oxidase (MAO) inhibitors, 220, 240
Moodswing (Fieve), 243–244
Moruzzi, Giuseppe, 172
Musès, Charles, 47–48
Mysticism, xi, 52

Nagylaki, Thomas, 129
Nerve functions, early beliefs about, 126–128
Neuroanatomy, 262
Neurobiology, and reality, 144–147
Neurochemistry, 262
  beginnings of, 216–217
Neurogenesis, 262
Neurons, 78, 82–83
  excitable membrane of, 84–85
  properties of, 84–86
  and sensory information, 86–87
Neuropsychology, 112–123
Neuroscience, 53
Neurosurgery, 162–173
Neurotransmitter, 85, 218–220
  acetylcholine, 219
  catecholamines, 218
  serotonin, 218–219
Neville, Robert C., 155–156
Nietzsche, Friedrich, 64
Nixon, Richard M., 257, 258
Noetics, 47–48
Nutritional therapy, 227–236

Ommaya, Ayub, 156
Operant conditioning, 185
ORG 2766 (synthetic ACTH), 96

Orthomolecular therapy, 227–236
  claims to therapies of, 234–235
  and orthodox neurochemistry, 232–233
Orthonoia, 52
Osmond, J. Humphrey, 231–232
Out-of-the-body (OOB) projection, 60

Paranoia, 52
Paraphysics, 53–54
Parapsychological Association, 61
Parapsychology, 58
Parkinsonism, 164, 165–167, 222–223
  stereotaxis for, 153–154
Parloff, Morris, 179–180, 181–195
Pauling, Linus, 229, 233–234
Pavlov, Ivan, 127
Pearce, Joseph Chilton, 55
Pellagra, 231
Perception, 262
Pettigrew, Jack, 141
Pfeiffer, Carl, 230, 232, 233
Phenylketonuria, 230
Piaget, Jean, 119
Pineal gland, x
Pinel, Philippe, 177–178
Pines, Maya, 90–100
Pituitary gland, 87
Plant communication, 54
Polarity therapy, 50
Political power, and mental illness, 246–260
Poltergeists, 60
Pratt, Fletcher, 70
Precognition, 59
Preventive psychiatry, 212–213
Primal therapy, 192–193
Psi movement, 4, 5
  meaning of, 57–58

Psi movement *(cont'd)*
  layman's guide to, 57–61
Psychenaut program, 17–26
Psychiatry, 178–180
  invasion of public affairs, 248–249
  limits of, 259–260
  and political power, 246–260
  practitioners' biases, 196–197
  preventive, 211–214
  and social class and race, 195–198
Psychic energy, 54
Psychic healing, 60
Psychic research, 54–55
  background of, 58
  definition of, 57
Psychic surgery, 60
Psychoanalysis, 178–180, 199–210
  analyst's role, 209
  in general culture, 206–208
  history and future of, 208–210
  long-distance, 250
  method of, 203–205
  revelation of, 201–202
  theory of, 205–208
  see also Psychiatry; Psychotherapy
Psychochemicals, 88
Psychoenergetics, 58
Psychokinesis (PK), 58, 59–60
Psychopharmacology, 239
Psychophysical education, 27–33
  and conventional physical education, 28–29
  and pleasure principle, 31
Psychopolitics, 252
Psychosurgery, 148–158
  amygdalotomies, 153
  cingulotomies, 153
  compared to brain surgery, xv
  ethics of, 150, 155–157
  lobotomy, 151–152
  need for research, 159–161

NIMH conference on, 149–150
  recommendations for monitoring, 157–158
  research results, 154–155
Psychosynthesis, 188
Psychotechnological medication, 252
Psychotherapy:
  analytically oriented, 183–184
  behavior therapy, 185–186
  group, 189–190
  humanistic, 186–187
  major schools of, 183
  pantheoretical approaches, 190–191
  role of therapist, 182, 195
  schools and techniques of, 181–195
  special treatment forms of, 189–193
  spectrum of, 177–180
  transpersonal, 187–189
  trends in, 193–194
  see also Psychiatry; Psychoanalysis
Psychotronics, 58
Puharich, Andrija, 51
Pure alexia without agraphia, 115–116, 123
Puromycin, 92–93
Puthoff, Harold, 54

Radical therapy, 190
Rama, Swami, 49
Reading-writing relation, 115–116
Reality:
  and the American Presidency, 256–259
  consensual, 146
  and culture, 146
  in humanistic therapy, 186–187
  and neurobiology, 144–147

Reality *(cont'd)*
  studies of, 55
Reflexes, and voluntary control, 40
Reich, Wilhelm, 50, 54
Reincarnation, 60–61
Relaxation:
  and biofeedback, 38–39
  progressive, 50
  techniques for, 50
Religion:
  and meditation research, 51–52
  and nature of man, 11
Reserpine, 219
Restak, Richard, 88, 101–111, 148–158, 159
Retrocognition, 59
Rhine, J.B., 57, 58
Rimland, Bernard, 233, 234–235
Ringsdorf, W.M., Jr., 229
RNA molecules, 82
Roberts, Jane, 55
Robinson, Frank M., 70
Robots, 67–70
  positronic, 67
Rodale, J.J., 229
Rodgers, Joann, 227–236
Rolf, Ida, 49–50
Rolfing, 49–50
Rosenfeld, Albert, ix–xvi, 3–6, 77–81, 82–87, 144–147, 159–161, 177–180, 211–214
Rozin, Paul, 123
Ruse, Gary Alan, 66

Saberhagen, Fred, 72
Sagan, Carl, 50
Sakitt, Barbara, 9
Schizophrenia, 221–222
  and diet, 228–229, 230
  heredity vs. environment, 225–226
  immunological aspects of, xv
  "true," as deficiency disease, 231–232

types of, 232
Schlesinger, Arthur, Jr., 246–260
Science fiction:
  and artificial intelligence, 65–70
  and evolution, 64–65
  mind-and-supermind in, 62–74
  relation to science, 64–65
  "wild talents" in, 70–71
Scott, Hugh, 258
Selesnick, Sheldon T., 178
Self-actualization, 56, 186–187
Self-consciousness, emergence of, 202
Self-control (biofeedback), 34–46
  site and precision of, 36–37
Self-image, 19, 120
Senile dementia, 234
Sensory acuity, 24–25
Sensory information, role of, 40–41
Sensory receptors, 83, 85–86
Sexism, 191
Shaw, George Bernard, 16, 64
Shelley, Mary, 64
Sherrington, Charles, 172
Silverman, Julian, 52
Situational crisis, 213–214
Skinner, B.F., 201, 251
Smith, Cordwainer, 69
Smith, Edward E., 73
Snow, C.P., 166
Sparks, Robert, 121
Sperry, Roger W., xii, 124–133
Spinelli, Nico, 140
Spirit photography, 60
Spirit possession, 60
Split-brain, 125–126
Steiner, Rudolf, 54
Stereotaxis, 153–154
Stevenson, George H., 249
Stimoceiver, 104–105
Stone, Randolph, 50

Structural integration (Rolfing), 49–50
Sturgeon, Theodore, 65
Subjective experience:
  and brain function, 131–133
  and eye movements, 134
Supermind, 3–4
Survival phenomena (theta), 58, 60–61
Sutich, Anthony, 56
Sweet, William, 171
Synapse, 85, 217–219
Synesthesia, 24
Szasz, Thomas, 179

Tanner, Charles R., 72
Tardive dyskinesia, 153
Targ, Russell, 54
Telekinesis, 59
Telepathy, 59
Teleportation, 59
Thalamus, 165
Thanatology, 55–56
Theta rhythm, 106
Thomas, Theodore L., 65
Thorazine, 153
Thoughtography, 60
Thudichum, J.W.L., 216–217
Tiller, William, 54
Time:
  acceleration of, 16–17
  compression of, 15–16, 23–24, 32
Torrey, E. Fuller, 179
Trance state, 15–17, 22
Tranquilizers, 153
  major, 222
Transactional analysis (TA), 189–190
Transcendental meditation (TM), 188–189
Transference, 201
The Transformation (Leonard), 12
Transformations, historical, 12–14

Transpersonal psychology, 56–57, 187–189

Ufology, 4, 50–51
Uncertainty principle, 101

Van den Bosch, F.J.G., 163n
Virus, 10
Vision:
  research on cats, 137–144
  visual-sensitive period, 141–144
Visual cortex, 138–141
Vitamin therapy, 227–236
Vogel, Philip, 125
Voltaire, François, 71
von Daniken, Erich, 50–51
von Euler, Ulf, 219
Vonnegut, Mark, 227–228, 230
von Weizsächer, C.F., 53

Waggoner, Raymond W., 249
War of the Worlds (Wells), 71–72
Watson, George, 229
Watson, John, 127–128
Watts, James, 151–152
Wechsler, James, 253
Weintraub, Karl, 202
Wells, H.G., 70, 71–72
White, John W., 47–57, 57–61, 267–272
Whorf, Benjamin Lee, 51, 119
Wiesel, Torsten, 138–139, 141
"Wild talents," 70–71
Wilde, Oscar, 207
Williamson, Jack, 67
Winograd, Terrence, 51
Wolff, Anthony, 237–245
Wyatt, Richard Jed, 236

Yoga, 30, 45
  Raja, 188
You Are Not Alone (Park-Shapiro), 274

Zurif, Edgar, 121